YogaPause

YogaPause

What Women Need to Know After 40 and Why Yoga is the Answer

Cheryl Kennedy MacDonald

YogaPause

Copyright © 2023 by Cheryl Kennedy MacDonald

All rights reserved. No part of this book may be reproduced or used in any manner without written permission of the copyright owner except for the use of quotations in a book review.

Dedicated to my wee mum,

with gratitude and love

Table of Contents

Introduction
    So, What Is YogaPause?
    Who Is It For?
    What Does It Cover?
1. The Importance of an Integrated Approach to Perimenopause
    Why Do I Need Yoga After 40?
    Understanding Perimenopause
2. The Science Bit: Hormones 101
    Adrenals and Perimenopause
    Hormone Basics
    Testing Your Hormones
3. Understanding the Symptoms and How to Manage Them
    Simple Modifications to Make to Your Yoga Practice After 40
    Your Menstrual Cycle in Perimenopause
    Charting and Tracking
    Aligning With The Lunar Phases In Menopause
4. Incorporating Yoga into Your Journey
    How to Develop a Yoga Practice that Works for You and Your Body
    The YogaPause Sadhana
5. Yoga to Help Tackle 'Fun' Perimenopause Challenges
    Insomnia and Sleep Disturbances

    Hot Flashes
    Menopausal Mood Madness
    Brain Fog
    Joint Pain
    Menorrhagia (Heavy Periods)
    Osteopenia and Bone Health
    Menopausal Middle and Weight Gain

6. An Extra Something: Incorporating Weights into Your Perimenopause Yoga Practice

7. Your Lovely Yoni (and it's a sad decline!)
    Natural Options for Vaginal Restoration
    Medication and Hormones
    Yoga for Your Vagina
    Let's Talk Yoni Eggs
    Yoni Steaming

8. PMS: Is It Getting Out of Hand?
    Yoga for PMS
    Meditation For PMS:
    Moon-time Journalling

9. Where's My Libido? Yoga, Orgasms and Your Sex Life in Perimenopause
    Let's Look at What Orgasms Can Do for You
    My Top Yoga Tips for Improving Your Sex Life Mid-Life
    Yoga and Meditation to Heighten Your Libido

10. Incorporating Yoga into Your Daily Routine

11. Happy Mind: Happy Life
    Ageing and the Patriarchy
    Everyday Mindfulness and Impermanence

Affirmations
   Sankalpa
12. Yoga and Positivity
   Why Does Yoga Make You Happy?
   Why is Oxytocin so important for women
   Why Getting Older Is Cool AF
13. Embracing the 'Enchantress' and 'Wise Woman' Phases of Life
   The Enchantress
   The Wise Woman
14. Strategies for overcoming challenges and sticking to your wellness practices
   Finding the support and resources that you need during perimenopause
15. Superfoods, Eating and The Right Nutrition for Optimal Health and Longevity
   Understanding the role of nutrition in staying fit and frisky
   Hormone-Happy Recommendations for a Balanced Diet
   Eat, Binge and Avoid
   Understanding food sensitivities and allergies and how they could impact your health.
   The Best Herbs, Supplements, and Minerals for the Menopause Journey
   Luscious Essential Oil Blends
16. Pause for Thought …
17. Hormone-Balancing Recipes
   Breakfast

    Snacks
    Lunchtime
    Dinnertime
    Desserts

18. Menopause Resources and Links

Bibliography

About the Author

Love this book? Check out the accompanying journal

Introduction

The first thing that I want to say is that I freaking love my forties! This has been my favourite decade so far, and I would not swap forty-three for twenty-three for all the money in the world. Seriously. That said, there are things that start happening around this age that nobody wants to talk about. We're hit with so many unexpected and undiscussed physical and emotional changes. Nobody ever sits you down to give you "the talk" about Menopause, and society dictates that we pretend it's not happening. Nobody wants to admit that they often look and feel like they've just eaten a very small chilli; that their hair is turning grey and that they would rather watch paint dry than have rampant sex.

It's confusing, overwhelming, and downright scary. I want to talk about *all* of this stuff. So many of us feel despondent, lost and utterly unsupported as we move into what should be an exciting and liberating phase of life: That's why I created YogaPause™. I want to show you why embracing yoga as a lifestyle can help you stay frisky, flexible, and fabulous throughout this rollercoaster of a journey. Yoga - on and off the mat - can help you prepare your body and mind for an optimal menopause, even if you're not quite there yet.

Contrary to popular belief, getting older does not mean that you suddenly cease to exist as a woman. Menopause is not The End. I promise you, that this can be the BEST time of your life. Free from the tyrant of menstrual biology and monthly hormonal madness; the huge commitment of caring for young children and being able to embrace your true self, possibly for the first time ever. This next stage of life has so much to offer.

My mum was in full-swing perimenopause in her early forties, so I knew I'd be around the same time. What I really remember about that time was that my mum was emotional and erratic. I had no idea what she was going through and I'm sure that my poor wee mum didn't have a clue either, but there was definitely a visible shift in her moods and behaviour that I noticed even at my young age.

If the information available now is scant, it was non-existent twenty years ago and NOBODY was openly talking about Menopause. The only thing I had ever heard about Menopause was when people would whisper things like, "oh she's going through the change," and that meant to me, that someone was becoming an old lady. Hot flashes were the only other thing that I knew was commonly associated with menopause, and I didn't really know what that was.

Introduction

Phrases like "dried up" and "past her prime" were (and still are) thrown around a lot too. So here we had this image of an angry, red faced, white haired little old lady storming around and that was the general consensus on menopause. You can see why the next phase of life was not warmly anticipated and was massively misunderstood by pretty much everyone.

The fact is that most of us start to move into perimenopause at some point after 35, even if the symptoms are imperceivable. This is because after our mid-thirties, our ovaries gradually begin to produce fewer hormones, (mainly oestrogen and progesterone,) which are important for regulating our menstrual cycle and reproductive health. So, although most of us know that our fertility begins to decline after thirty-five, we don't generally realise that this also means the beginning of perimenopause. This is especially true now, when so many of us are having babies in our late thirties and forties. I often meet women in class who've just given birth and shortly after this, have started experiencing perimenopause symptoms (this can be especially confusing as many postpartum symptoms mirror menopause symptoms, but more on that later.) Our hormone levels don't just immediately drop when perimenopause kicks in, they fluctuate a lot at this point, and this is when we might start to see 'symptoms' rear their ugly heads.

As I moved into my forties it occurred to me that I really had no idea what came next. I had just never really thought about life after motherhood. Being a busy working mum, I hadn't had five minutes to myself in the past decade, never mind had time to ponder getting old. I'm sure that many of you are in the same situation now, especially if you still have a young family. So, when my menstrual cycle started to become erratic AF and I started to experience persistent UTIs and thrush-like symptoms, I didn't immediately connect the dots or equate this as anything to do with perimenopause. It was not just not on my radar at all.

First stop was the GP. I went in with my myriad of lady complaints to get some antibiotics for my UTI. The antibiotics resulted in causing more discomfort and even gave me thrush. I was then given creams and tablets and pessaries for those symptoms. The UTI hadn't cleared up at all, in fact things were getting worse, so I went back to my GP looking for some different antibiotics and some answers. I was prescribed some new antibiotics, which resulted in some more thrush, but that was about it. I was going around in circles, becoming increasingly frustrated, in constant pain and getting nowhere. No connection was ever made between these symptoms and my irregular menstrual cycles and at no point was perimenopause mentioned. The clearly uninterested physicians (or perhaps they were just lacking in useful knowledge) never looked further than the obvious culprits and the basic prescription pad.

Now what I'm about to describe is highly unlikely to happen to most women, but I think it's important to share this with you, as it does show you the worst possible scenario. This is one extreme example of why you need to be aware of perimenopause. After six months of this situation getting progressively worse, the persistent UTIs turned into a kidney infection. I was doubled up in pain groaning and vomiting... and I was given more of the same antibiotics. A couple of days later, I went to A&E and was sent home. Three times. Eventually, I was admitted to hospital with Sepsis and came VERY close to dying. I was placed on intravenous antibiotics and was in intensive care for quite some time. So, from what we consider to be straight-forward female ailments, to a near death situation, is not great.

What's that got to do with perimenopause? Well, UTIs are more common during perimenopause because of declining oestrogen levels. This leads to changes in the urinary tract, making us more susceptible to infections. Oestrogen helps to keep the urinary tract healthy by keeping the tissues lubricated and preventing harmful bacteria. When oestrogen declines, the urinary tract becomes thinner and drier. As we get older, our immune system function also declines, making us even more susceptible to infections, like UTIs. Women over forty with UTIs and other reproductive symptoms need to be thinking about the possibility of perimenopause, as these conditions are often related. I should have been given further testing at the outset, like blood tests to measure my hormone levels or a pelvic exam, to evaluate for perimenopause or other gynaecological conditions. However, the common conception - even in medical circles - is that menopause only happens to 'older women,' so it wasn't picked up. If it had been, this would have helped me get the appropriate treatment and identified any underlying hormonal imbalances, and possibly have saved me from this grim experience.

This is one reason why it's so important for us to understand what perimenopause is: So that we know what's really going on in our bodies. Then we can get started ASAP on giving our bodies what they need now, which is not the same as what they needed in our twenties. Then we can seek out the help and support that we need when these seemingly 'minor' things happen. Medics and the general public just don't know enough about menopause and women everywhere are suffering because nobody will help them or even acknowledge what they're going through.

This was a particularly ropey start to my forties, but I promise you that it got and continues to get a whole lot better. When I recovered from Sepsis, I started to explore the menopause journey in the same way that I had immersed myself in all thing's pregnancy and baby in my twenties to create YogaBellies (hello

Introduction

hyperfocus!) I was utterly compelled to explore this new phase of life: The good bits, the bad bits and what I could do to make it better for myself and to support other women. I just knew that yoga was going to be the answer, just as it had supported me through every other life transition. Over the past few years, I've absorbed every single bit of information I could get my hands on; every scientific fact; every holistic practice and yoga technique that could be useful to help my fellow menopause traveller. You're going to find it all in this book.

N.B. You may be wondering why I'm writing about *Perimenopause* and not *Menopause*. There's a common misconception that when you start to get symptoms like hot flashes and irregular periods that THIS is Menopause. In fact, Menopause is technically only one single day: The date is exactly one year or 12 months from when you had your last menstrual period. So, everything leading up to that - the ups and downs, the symptoms and the chaos - all of this is really 'Perimenopause.' From the beginning of perimenopause to post-menopause, it is all part of the 'menopause journey.'

So, What Is YogaPause?

I want to share my personal journey and the yoga practices, tools and rituals that I've used to improve my mental health, fitness and lust for life after 40, and used to support hundreds of other women on the same journey. Basically, what keeps bringing me back to yoga; how it has carried me to my glorious forties and why it is the solution to absolutely everything.

YogaPause approaches this cracking new life stage by combining yoga, fitness, nutrition and self-care and most importantly, focuses on establishing a positive ageing mindset. You need all of these things and more to live a whole and happy life, and I'm going to give you practical, easy-to-follow advice that will make a big difference. I'll also provide options to help you design your personalised yoga and lifestyle plan, manage your libido and sexual health, and balance your hormones. Boom!

Who Is It For?

All women over thirty-five, that's who! If you go to an occasional yoga class or thought, yep, now is the time to start yoga (all the hot forty-plus celebs do, after all) then welcome! If that's the case, you may still be thinking of yoga in terms of the physical stuff or perhaps you've heard about the more calming and meditative aspects of the practice. All of this is valuable and true, and I will of course cover that, but I'd also like to explain why yoga can make a huge impact on how you experience life. Yoga can be a lifestyle and should be integrated into *every* aspect of your life, on and off the yoga mat. A way of looking at

Introduction

every experience you have; how you function in the *right now* and how you react to people and situations. It's a whole vibe.

You could, on the other hand, be an experienced yogini with thousands of hours of yoga teacher training under your belt and this is for you too. I want to also remind anyone reading this book to note that I am not a medical professional. Please be sure to discuss with your physician, any new diet, yoga, or holistic practice that you may want to try. I am a Yoga and Meditation Master and hold my post-grad in Psychotherapy and Counselling. I am a Meditation Guide, Naturopath, Aromatherapist, Yoni Steam Practitioner, Tantric Priestess and hold many more weird and wonderful titles from my myriad of training over the years. What you will get from this book is my almost three-decade yoga journey and how that has supported me and the women I've worked with. I've provided a bibliography containing the sources for all the information in this book at the end, if you want to dive deeper into any specific area.

From the spiritual to the bendy to the downright weird, you'll find in here *what I believe yoga to be* and how it has helped me personally. I hope that you find tools and tips in here that help you too.

What Does It Cover?

I've included YogaPause practices to try at home to help alleviate some of the most common menopause symptoms. I've also provided meditations and affirmations to work alongside your physical yoga practice. We'll also look at the option of incorporating light weights into your yoga practice and why this can be a good choice for women as they age.

You'll also find some 'yoni-focused practices,' like yoni yoga and working with jade eggs and vaginal steaming. Lots of exotic but useful advice from me on keeping your yoni happy and healthy, long past menopause. (FYI Yoni is Sanskrit for vulva, referring to it as a symbol of divine procreative energy.) N.B. I am NOT against HRT (Hormone Replacement Therapy), and we'll peek at this too. I've only discussed HRT with regards to vaginal atrophy, but there are tons of resources out there for more detailed information on the broader scope of HRT options and I recommend that you do look at this option too.

We'll explore embracing positivity and why yoga really does make you happy and is the solution to a long and happy life. We'll look at living mindfully, reducing your stress levels, and integrating simple yoga practices into your daily routine. Making tiny, incremental lifestyle changes can have a huge impact on your health and happiness.

I'll also introduce you to the two Goddess archetypes most connected to the menopause journey: The

Introduction

Enchantress and the Wise Woman. I'll explain the power of welcoming these archetypes into your life throughout menopause and I'll provide you with meditations and yoga practices to help you channel your inner Goddess.

Something you may have overlooked until now is nutrition. It's boring and we like chocolate and that's not about to change now, right? It's a bit more complicated than that as we get older, with the wrong foods causing a lot more problems for us and the right ones giving us the energy we need to keep going. I want to explore our relationship with food and also, with our weight as we age. We'll discover what foods we should be eating and those to avoid and how this could all change. We'll look at herbs and supplements that can help, and at the end of the book, you'll find a ton of tasty, hormone-balancing recipes that contain all the nutrients you need for the menopause journey.

As the founder of YogaBellies™, I've worked with women at every stage of life. I've seen first-hand how yoga can be a powerful tool for managing hormonal fluctuations, improving bone density, and alleviating symptoms like hot flashes, mood swings, and insomnia. I've experienced myself how a positive ageing mindset (I call it PAM) and these simple lifestyle changes can make all the difference to how we feel and look.

This book is not just about managing the symptoms of perimenopause with yoga, but about empowering you to take control of your health and your life as you move past your thirties. With the right approach and frame of mind, it is possible to absolutely live your best life and keep doing so, far beyond Menopause. Whether you are just beginning your journey or are well into it, I've written this book to provide you with all the knowledge, resources, and tools you need to thrive.

The 10 Menopause Mysteries: Things Most Commonly Misunderstood About Menopause

Let's start with the things that are most commonly unknown or misunderstood about life after 40 or the 'menopause mysteries,' as I call them:

1. Perimenopause can start years before menopause: Many women don't realise that it can start several years before menopause, most often in our late 30s or early 40s. One of the very first signs can be changes in the length or heaviness of your menstrual cycle. Even if you've had a baby in your forties, this doesn't mean that you're not in perimenopause.

2. It's a natural process, not a disease: Perimenopause happens as our hormones start to shift in preparation for menopause. It's not an illness, and there's no need to be alarmed or

embarrassed by the symptoms and there are remedies and solutions to help.

3. Symptoms can be diverse: Perimenopause can cause a wide range of symptoms, including hot flashes, night sweats, mood swings, irritability, fatigue, sleep disturbances, and more. Your friend's experience may be completely different from yours and that's ok.

4. Hormonal changes are a major cause of the issue: As oestrogen levels fluctuate and decline, this can lead to fluctuations in other hormones, leading to those pleasant symptoms I just described.

5. It can impact sexual function: Perimenopause can also impact your sex life and function, stemming from fun side-effects such as making your vagina as dry as old toast, pain during intercourse, and decreased libido.

6. Perimenopause and menopause are not the same thing: Perimenopause is the transition (and the symptoms that we hear about) to Menopause. Menopause is defined as 12 months after the last menstrual period and the permanent end of menstrual cycles. Everything past this point is then post-menopause.

7. Menopause is technically only one day BUT it is not a one-time event: Menopause does not happen suddenly, but rather it's a process that occurs over several years. Before the cycles stop, this is known

as Perimenopause. 'Menopause' is a journey through all of these stages.

8. Hormone replacement therapy is not the only option but it's often a good option: While hormone replacement therapy can help to relieve symptoms, lifestyle changes such as diet, exercise (Yoga!), and stress management, can also be very effective in managing your symptoms. However, you don't just have to rely on one or the other: I believe that an integrated approach to menopause is best.

9. It's still possible to get pregnant: While perimenopause marks the transition to menopause, it's still possible to get pregnant during this time, so don't ditch the pills and condoms just yet. Many a mama has been caught out this way!

10. There are now resources available: Many of us don't realise that there are a growing number of resources available to help us manage our symptoms and navigate this time of life. From healthcare providers to yoga classes and support groups, to online resources, there's help there if you need it, Chica!

1. The Importance of an Integrated Approach to Perimenopause

Perimenopause is a complex time. We're experiencing changes that are impacting not only our health, but our whole lives and our way of looking at the world. The symptoms and even the societal aspects can be downright challenging, but there are tons of strategies and tools that can make managing this transition a little bit easier.

One of the best ways to tackle perimenopause, as I said, is with an integrated approach. This means incorporating medical, non-medical and holistic tools into your menopause kit bag. I'll touch upon each of these, and how they can work together for the best outcomes.

Yoga. I'm going to talk about this a lot, but it has been my absolute saviour at every life stage. Yoga will help to increase your physical strength, flexibility, and balance, as well as reducing your levels of stress and anxiety. This ancient and awesome practice can also help regulate hormonal imbalances and in turn, lessen menopause symptoms.

Nutrition is another important aspect of your wellness we'll look at. Eating a balanced, nutrient-dense diet can help support healthy hormone levels, reduce inflammation, and boost your (flagging) energy levels. Making mindful food choices are an important key to our health as we get older.

Having a positive mindset around ageing is an incredibly powerful, if not essential tool. This means cultivating a pro-ageing outlook, setting yourself realistic and achievable life goals, and learning to cope with stress and anxiety in healthy ways (i.e., not hitting the Sav Blanc every night). By cultivating the right frame of mind, we can better manage our physical and emotional symptoms and stay in tip-top condition so that we can keep being our fabulous selves.

By incorporating all these things into your new approach to life, you can take control of your health and thrive during this brilliant, if somewhat confusing, life phase.

Why Do I Need Yoga After 40?

The number of women who begin practising yoga after the age of forty is on the continual rise, with women realising that yoga is *the* way to reduce the discomforts and unpleasantries associated with menopause and ageing. As a yoga teacher, I've personally seen the number of women over forty coming to yoga, double over the past ten years.

The benefits that can be reaped from yoga are far higher for women than men, as we tend to experience hormonal fluctuations throughout life. The hormonal changes in menopause are the same hormones affecting us during menstruation, often causing PMS. That's why a lot of what you're feeling may not feel so unfamiliar.

So, how can yoga help women during menopause?

If you're not practising yoga after 40, you are doing yourself a complete disservice. It lowers stress: Yoga controls breathing, which reduces anxiety. It also clears all of those negative feelings and thoughts, reducing the chance of suffering from depression. It's a proven effective method to reduce and control your anger, often referred to as 'Menorage,' something else that may be exacerbated by hormonal fluctuations. If you are practising yoga regularly, your overall sense of 'life is good' will increase, making life a little less stressful and a lot more fun.

It eases physical pain and discomfort. Yoginis are known to have higher pain tolerance. Aches and pains associated with perimenopause can be alleviated along with things like back pain, or other chronic pain such as neck or joint pain. It doesn't have to be fancy either. A simple, gentle yoga practice like a flowing *Surya Namaskara* (sun salutations) will help to increase flexibility in your joints and work every muscle in your body. It's a complete physical and emotional workout in itself. Try practising 5–10 rounds a day, even if you don't have time for any other yoga, you will experience some dramatic relief from body aches.

It decreases the hassles of hot flushes. During perimenopause, hot flushes are caused by an excess of *pitta* (which in Ayurveda means fire) in the body, and that has to come out! There are specific *asanas* (yoga postures which we'll discuss later), which can help, as well as breathing practices. Movements should be slow and weight-bearing, paying close attention to the rhythm of the breath and the position of the tongue to the roof of the palate during practice. This allows the mind to become calm and stabilise.

It reduces blood pressure. A common symptom during menopause is night sweats. Regular yoga practice reduces high blood pressure and promotes oxygenation and blood circulation in the body, which helps lessen the frequency and severity of the terrible night sweats. *Savasana* (corpse pose) is perfect for allowing yourself to relax and just bring your attention to the breath. By taking our focus away from the stresses and strains of the outside world, we can focus on what's happening right now, helping to alleviate anxieties.

It's a natural remedy. Yoga is a fantastic and natural way to help alleviate pain associated with changes in the menstrual cycle. So many women suffer in silence or take endless pills, but yoga is an ideal way to soothe these symptoms. Cramps, heavy flow, back ache and migraines can all be helped with the right yoga practice.

Yoga is even better when combined with aromatherapy. Not only are your senses enthralled by the beautiful aromas during your practice, but the focus and effects of your practice are also intensified by the therapeutic use of essential oil blends. Healing benefits of aromatherapy oils include releasing old or negative emotions; experiencing a detoxifying or cleansing feeling; soothing tense muscles; helping to balance hormonal fluctuations or even helping to realign the chakras and promote feelings of calm and peace. I've included some beautiful blends you can try later on in the book.

It is great for the joints. Yoga has been proven time and time again to help people suffering from problems associated with joints, such as arthritis. While not all menopausal women will have arthritis, it's a health concern that's often associated with ageing. Research shows that practising *hatha* (physical) yoga can help to ease joint pain, fatigue, and other related symptoms. The small study involved women aged 21 to 35 that on average had suffered from rheumatoid arthritis for 10 and a half years. After six weeks, they asked both groups about their condition. The group that practised yoga said they were happier than when they started and could better accept and manage their pain. The women were also reported to have better general health and more energy in general.

A big fan of YogaBellies and a lady who experienced the benefits of yoga for menopause first-hand was Jo Dunn who runs Bosom Buddies, a bra fitting service in Glasgow. At age 53, her first symptoms kicked in: Her mood dropped, she felt anxious and woke up every night with dreadful night sweats. Despite trying several herbal remedies, the symptoms showed no signs of slowing down, and after meeting Cheryl from YogaBellies, Jo decided to give yoga a try.

This is what Jo said: 'I'd heard yoga was a good way of learning to focus and relax with the added benefit of toning up the body and helping to cope with the menopause symptoms, but I didn't realise quite how effective it would be! It was so good to know I could help ease menopause without having to take tablets. It allowed me to feel more in control of the changes happening to my body.'

'When the menopause began, my waist seemed to disappear, and my confidence decreased. After just a few sessions, I started toning up again and began looking forward to going to work again. Not only has it helped the symptoms such as night sweats, but it's also made me sleep better and helped with physical problems which I've had for many years such as pains in my hips and knees. I'd highly recommend yoga to any woman experiencing menopausal symptoms.'

Understanding Perimenopause

Perimenopause is all about moving from our reproductive years into menopause. This transition can last anywhere from a few years to as long as a decade, and it's marked by the plethora of random symptoms we're going to explore. Fluctuations in hormone levels, changes in menstrual patterns and the onset of other surprises such as hot flashes, mood swings, and sleep disturbances, all make for good times ahead ladies!

We need to remember that perimenopause is a normal and natural part of the ageing process and that it is not a disease or disorder. However, it's nothing to be ashamed of and you don't need to deny it's happening, in fact, you absolutely should talk about it! There is no denying that hormonal and physiological changes can have a profound impact on our physical and emotional health, and it's important to be armed with a tool kit of knowledge and strategies so that you are fully prepared for any challenges that crop up.

As I mentioned, perimenopause symptoms are caused by fluctuations in hormone levels, namely, oestrogen, progesterone and the other hormones that regulate the menstrual cycle. As we head towards menopause, these hormones decline, leading to a decline in our fertility and the onset of symptoms.

Perimenopause can be challenging of course, but it can also be an awesome opportunity for growth, self-discovery and increasing self-care. In the following chapters, we'll explore the key components of an integrated approach to perimenopause, including what's actually going on; yoga I've created for this very life stage; nutritional advice; all of those juicy self-care practices and how to develop a goddess mindset. By bringing these practices into your daily routine, you can live a longer, happier, and more fulfilling life.

2. The Science Bit: Hormones 101

Okay the science bit. Straight biology may not be the most exciting of topics so feel free to skip this section if you genuinely know it all or find it as dry as a bone. However, I would encourage everyone to check this out, so that you absolutely understand what's going on inside. It's going to help you identify symptoms and understand where all of these strange changes are coming from.

These hormones that are currently up, down and diminishing at a rapid speed, are the same hormones that affected us when we started to menstruate, or you may recognise some of them from looking into menstrual disorders or from when you were pregnant.

Adrenals and Perimenopause

When hormone production drops in the ovaries, the adrenal glands take over. At the same time, the adrenals continue producing testosterone, cortisol, and adrenaline, which allow us to deal with the ongoing stressors of the day. The severity of symptoms experienced during perimenopause like hot flashes, trouble sleeping, and mood swings are influenced by the production of those hormones by the adrenals.

Often, symptoms of perimenopause can look like adrenal fatigue symptoms. If you find yourself constantly stressed and have fatigue, trouble sleeping, weight gain, moodiness or mental fogginess, there is a chance that you could actually be experiencing adrenal fatigue instead of thinking you're in the perimenopause stage of life. This is where the DUTCH test can come in very handy, but you have to find a practitioner who can interpret it.

If you're a 50-year-old woman that is rarely stressed out and you suddenly start having hot flashes, feeling anxious and experiencing trouble sleeping, most likely, you're entering perimenopause. Whereas if you're 25 years old and you start feeling fatigued, anxious, etc, you may want to check your adrenal health.

Hormone Basics

Oestrogen

The female body makes three major types of oestrogen.

1. Oestradiol (E2) is the most abundant form of oestrogen in women of childbearing years. E2 is important for maintaining regular menstrual cycles and for overall health.

2. Estriol (E3) is only detected in significant quantities during pregnancy because it is produced by the placenta.

3. Estrone (E1) is the main oestrogen produced after menopause.

- Oestrogen not only plays a critical role in regulating menstruation and reproduction, but it is also key for neurological processes, bone growth, cholesterol levels, urinary tract, heart and blood vessels, skin, hair, mucous membranes, and pelvic muscles.

- Oestrogen tests are used to detect imbalance. The levels of each type of oestrogen in conjunction with information about your cycle can aid in diagnosing conditions associated with an imbalance.

Progesterone

Progesterone is important in preparing the body for pregnancy. Each menstrual cycle, after the egg is released, the corpus luteum releases progesterone, and progesterone levels dramatically increase. This hormone prepares the lining of the uterus for fertilised eggs to attach and prevents the uterine lining from shedding if an egg is fertilised. If the egg is not fertilised, progesterone levels decrease, and the lining sheds. This shedding is what causes menstrual bleeding.

- During pregnancy, progesterone levels should remain high, so the placenta grows, and the foetus is nourished.

- In perimenopause, progesterone tests help your doctor assess ovulatory function.

Testosterone

Testosterone may be thought of as a male hormone, but women need testosterone for bone strength, cognitive performance, and a healthy sex drive. Women with inadequate levels of testosterone experience low libido and are at higher risk of osteoporosis. Too much testosterone in women can cause the development of excess body hair, facial hair, and acne; PCOS and a higher risk of infertility can also result.

Follicle-stimulating And Luteinizing hormones

Follicle-stimulating hormone (FSH) is released by the pituitary gland. FSH stimulates the follicles in your ovaries to mature. The pituitary gland then releases Luteinizing Hormone (LH), which is responsible for ovulation. Only one follicle will "ripen" and become mature during each cycle.

- Tests for FSH and LH are used to check fertility and to predict when a woman will naturally enter menopause.

Cortisol

Cortisol is a stress hormone. It is released by the adrenal glands, and it impacts digestion and hunger, sleeping and waking, blood pressure, insulin, immunity, and inflammatory response, as well as our stress response.

- A cortisol test is used to check cortisol levels and to diagnose disorders of the adrenal glands. Because stress can play such a big part in sex hormone production, checking cortisol can help your practitioner get a more well-rounded picture of your health and hormone status.

Thyroid Hormones

Because so many symptoms of perimenopause overlap thyroid imbalance, it can be a good idea to check thyroid hormone levels.

- The three main thyroid hormones to test are TSH, free T3 and free T4.
- TSH is a hormone made by the pituitary gland that stimulates the thyroid to make hormones. If the pituitary gland is producing abnormally high levels of TSH, it may mean that your thyroid gland is not making enough hormones. On its own, TSH does not tell us about the health of the thyroid.
- T4 is the main hormone produced by the thyroid. It is inactive until conversion in the liver to T3.

By testing TSH, free T3 and free T4, your practitioner can assess if your thyroid is producing enough hormone and if your body is converting T4 to the active/usable form (T3).

rT3 is another useful test. This measures the amount of reverse T3 which is an inactive form of T3. The body converts T3 to rT3 when it notes an excess of T3.

Sometimes, this conversion can happen in error or excess. rT3 binds to the same receptors as T3, so too much of this hormone can prevent T3 from getting into your cells. This can be a helpful piece of information if your thyroid labs otherwise look normal, but you're experiencing symptoms of being hypothyroid.

Testing Your Hormones

No single test can determine if you've entered perimenopause. There are other things to consider, including age, menstrual history and the symptoms or body changes you're experiencing.

The important thing to know is that testing only reflects your hormone levels on the day of testing. Hormones shift during your cycle and can be impacted by hormonal birth control, hormone replacement therapy and some meds. Some supplements, such as biotin(B7), can also interfere with hormone tests such as TSH, FSH, LH, T4, T3, Oestradiol, Testosterone and Cortisol.

The following home testing kits are also available:

- Everlywell Perimenopause Test
- myLAB Box Perimenopause Test

If you're working with a practitioner, these labs may be helpful:

- Follicle-stimulating hormone
- Luteinizing hormone
- Oestradiol
- Testosterone

If you have a practitioner who is trained in reading the DUTCH test, it can provide valuable information about hormones and adrenals as well. Please talk with your physician about any questions or concerns you have about testing options and/or the best timing for testing.

IF YOU ARE CURRENTLY TAKING HORMONES

Testing will accurately reflect your 'current' hormone levels. If you're currently taking bioidentical or synthetic hormones, your hormone levels will change once you discontinue use. Many labs do not advise specific tests, such as ovarian function tests while taking hormone therapy (including hormonal birth control). I do not advise altering your hormone therapy without consulting your physician first. If discontinuing hormone therapy, labs recommend waiting six weeks until collecting the sample.

3. Understanding the Symptoms and How to Manage Them

What kind of symptoms and health challenges do we commonly experience during perimenopause?

A quick refresher on some of the main culprits:

Hot flashes: This is a common and well-known symptom of perimenopause. A hot flash is a sudden and intense feeling of warmth that spreads through the body, often accompanied by sweating and flushing of the skin.

Mood swings: Perimenopause can also cause mood swings, with feelings of irritability, anxiety and depression being quite common.

Sleep disturbances: Many women find that they have trouble sleeping during perimenopause, with symptoms like insomnia and night sweats.

Weight gain: Hormonal changes during perimenopause can cause changes in metabolism, leading to weight gain and difficulty losing weight.

Vaginal dryness: Perimenopause can cause changes in oestrogen levels, leading to dryness downstairs and discomfort during sex.

Fatigue: Many women experience feelings of exhaustion and low energy levels during perimenopause.

Brain fog: A decline in oestrogen levels can also cause brain fog, making it difficult to concentrate and remember things.

Changes in your libido: Some women experience a decreased interest in sex and others experience an increase!

It's important to understand that these symptoms are completely natural, and they will mostly eventually pass. However, they can be quite challenging to deal with in the meantime, so let's look at tackling these bad boys.

Let's start with some universal basic tips that you can apply right now. 'Perimenopause 101', if you will:

- Move regularly: Regular physical activity can help to reduce the severity of hot flashes, improve your mood, and regulate your weight.

- Eat a healthy diet: Practice mindful eating and focus on whole, nutrient-dense foods can help to manage weight, improve your energy levels, and improve your health overall.

- Practice stress management techniques: Yoga, mindfulness and deep breathing can help to reduce anxiety and depression.

- Get enough sleep: Aim for 7–9 hours of sleep every night, and avoid caffeine, alcohol, and electronics before bedtime.

- Seek treatment if necessary: If you're struggling with severe symptoms of perimenopause, it may be helpful to seek treatment from a healthcare professional. Hormonal therapies and other medications can help to manage symptoms but be sure to discuss your options with your doctor.

By taking a proactive and integrated approach, you can minimise the impact of these symptoms. In the next chapters, we'll talk about how yoga, nutrition and a positive mindset can help you to manage the challenges of perimenopause, so stay tuned.

Simple Modifications to Make to Your Yoga Practice After 40

Here are some basic modifications you can make to your yoga practice right now. Think of these simple pointers as a 'cheat sheet' to help you get the most out of your practice while staying safe and comfortable. Again, this applies to newbies and yoga experts alike. Always stay mindful of what your body is telling you it needs, right now.

Try gentle yoga postures: If you are focusing on managing symptoms, it helps to choose gentle yoga postures that are low impact and don't put too much strain on your body. For example, seated postures like Child's Pose, Forward Folds and Cobra Pose are great options.

Avoid inversions: During perimenopause, it is common to experience fluctuations in blood pressure, which can make us feel lightheaded or dizzy. To avoid any potential issues, I think it's best to avoid inversions like Headstands and Shoulder Stand. Instead, opt for postures that keep your head below your heart, like Downward Facing Dog and Cat-Cow. Of course, if you've been standing on your hands for years and want to keep doing this and it feels right carry on!

Pay attention to your breathing: Stress levels can be high because of those wild hormonal fluctuations. Practising deep, slow breathing can help to calm your mind and reduce that stress. In your yoga practice, take time to focus on your breath and make sure you're breathing deeply and fully. Always try to join the breath with the movement which is one of the ways that yoga becomes a moving meditation and not just another gym class.

Incorporate restorative yoga postures: Restorative yoga postures are designed to help you relax and rejuvenate your body. As we get older, it's important to prioritise self-care and rest. Try incorporating postures like Supported Child's Pose, Reclining Bound Angle Pose and Legs Up the Wall into your practice to help you feel refreshed and relaxed. If you've had a very dynamic practice (perhaps Ashtanga or Hot yoga) up until now, consider changing this up or at least introducing a restorative practice too.

Use props: You may start to experience physical limitations that make certain yoga postures more challenging than they were before, or you may want to slow the pace of your practice down. Things like props like blocks, heat packs, straps and weighted blankets can be incredibly helpful. They can provide support and make postures more accessible, allowing you to keep getting the most out of your practice. It's time to release the ego and enjoy using props, there's no shame in feeling comfortable. Play around with different props and adaptations and see what feels right.

Remember, the most important thing is to listen to your body and make modifications that work for you. Your yoga practice should be a source of comfort and relaxation, not a source of stress or discomfort. So, be gentle with yourself, and don't be afraid to make changes as needed to ensure your yoga practice is still giving you what you need.

Your Menstrual Cycle in Perimenopause

Let's explore what happens to your menstrual cycle now and what you can expect. For many women, the very first sign of the transition is a change in their menstrual cycle. This could look like:

Irregular periods: They may become more random, with longer or shorter cycles, or you may skip periods altogether.

Heavier or lighter periods: You may notice changes in the flow, with heavier or lighter bleeding than usual.

Spotting: Some women experience light bleeding or spotting in between periods.

Changes in your PMS symptoms: Your premenstrual symptoms, such as cramping, bloating, or mood changes may become more or less severe. (Check out my sequence for worsening PMS symptoms later in the book.)

Keep in mind that everyone's experience with perimenopause is different, so you may not see all of these changes, or you may experience them to a greater or lesser degree than someone else. It is all normal.

The changes to your menstrual cycle during perimenopause are natural. While they may be inconvenient at times, they are simply a sign that your body is transitioning to this new phase.

Charting and Tracking

Your cycle is going to undergo some serious irregularity and changes during perimenopause. One of the best ways to help predict your ovulation and bleeding days is to track them.

Remember, menopause only becomes official when you have not had a period in 12 months. Tracking your cycle can help you see when you enter perimenopause and then menopause, so you can start to prepare your body and mind and have a conversation about potential support options.

Aligning With The Lunar Phases In Menopause

So, basically, keeping up with the cycle of the moon can be really helpful for us as we go through the menopause journey. Our bodies are naturally designed to follow a monthly rhythm, and women's bodies especially are tuned in to this cycle. When our periods become irregular or stop altogether, if you haven't already, it's a good idea to sync up with the moon's tempo.

The time between one New Moon and the next is about 29.5 days, which is similar to the timing of a fertile woman's cycle. Our emotions also ebb and flow in a similar way. We feel like we're starting fresh at the end of our period, kind of like how a New Moon

Understanding the Symptoms and How to Manage Them

symbolizes a new beginning. After our period, our bodies start getting ready for pregnancy, and the moonlight starts to increase as it moves toward the Full Moon. Then, we ovulate at the Full Moon, and after that, our energy starts to decrease, much like how we feel during our period.

While standard calendars do follow a similar monthly pattern, they don't really align with the energetic and natural movements of the moon. Calendar months are just units of time with no real energy behind them. The first day of the month isn't any different energetically from the middle or end of the month. So, it's important to pay attention to the moon cycle to really cleanse and nourish our bodies.

You can start following the Moon cycle at any time. Each Moon phase has its own unique vibe and energy. But if you're a woman going through the stages of menopause and want to get in sync with this nurturing rhythm, the best time to start is during the Dark and New Moons, which actually reflect the perimenopause and menopause stages of a woman's life (more on this when we look at the wild woman and crone archetypes.)

The Dark Moon is the end of the cycle and comes a few days before the New Moon. It's a signal to rest and take it easy, so listen to your body and slow down if you're feeling tired. It's okay to take a break and enjoy nature's pause.

Women tend to sync more naturally with each other in modern society, rather than the Moon. However, if you don't have a strong sisterhood or group of close female friends, the Moon can be a great companion.

As the Dark Moon comes to an end, pay attention to any internal energy shifts. If you've rested properly, you may notice a natural arising of refreshed lightness and increased optimism, energy, and enthusiasm.

Take some time to observe the Dark and New Moons over a few months. Moonplay is a cumulative process, so you need to watch the Moon over time to get into the rhythm. Observing Full Moons is also beneficial, so try to notice how the days before, during, and after the Full Moon week differ from those of the Dark week. Tune into your body and describe what you feel in your journal, even if it's subtle. Over time, your sensitivity and discernment will increase.

Entraining to Moon phases can benefit all women, including premenopausal women, women without strong communities, and those who work full time outside the home. The corporate rhythm can be very masculine and tear us away from our instinctive feminine self.

Syncing your menstrual cycle with the lunar phases during perimenopause and menopause can be a great way to tap into the nurturing universal rhythm and find balance during this transition period. Even if your periods are irregular or have stopped altogether, you can still use the Moon as a guide to help you connect with nature and your own body.

Here are some tips on how to align your menstrual cycle with the lunar phases during perimenopause and menopause:

Observe the Moon: Take some time to notice the Moon's phases and how they make you feel. Now, even if you're not menstruating regularly anymore, you can still use the Lunar cycle as a guide. Start by paying attention to how the different phases of the Moon make you feel. The lunar cycle lasts around 29.5 days, so it's helpful to have a lunar calendar, moon phase journal or app to track the phases. The New Moon is the beginning of the lunar cycle, followed by the Waxing Moon, Full Moon, and Waning Moon. Each phase has its own unique energy and can help you connect with different aspects of yourself.

Sync with the Dark and New Moons: The Dark Moon, which comes a few days before the New Moon, is a time of rest and introspection. This is a great time to slow down and take care of yourself. The New Moon is a time of new beginnings, fresh starts, and setting intentions. It's a great time to focus on what you want to bring into your life.

Use the Full Moon for release: The Full Moon is a time of culmination and release. This is a great time to let go of what no longer serves you and make space for new things to come in. You can do a Full Moon ritual or simply take some time to reflect on what you want to release. Process by writing down what you want to let go of, and then burning or burying the paper as a symbolic act of release.

Align your self-care with the lunar phases: During the Waxing Moon, focus on self-care practices that support growth and expansion. This could include trying new things, taking a class, or starting a new project. During the Waning Moon, focus on self-care practices that support rest and relaxation. This could include taking a bath, meditating, or getting a massage.

Listen to your body: While it's helpful to use the Moon as a guide, it's also important to listen to your own body. Perimenopause and menopause can bring many changes to your body, and your menstrual cycle may no longer be a reliable indicator of your fertility or hormonal fluctuations. Instead, pay attention to how you feel and adjust your self-care practices accordingly.

Remember, syncing your menstrual cycle with the lunar phases is not about perfection or strict adherence to a specific schedule. It's about using the natural rhythms of the Moon to support your own personal growth and well-being during this transition period. It's such a beautiful way to connect with the natural rhythms of the universe and your body and we discuss the lunar phases and their relevance to our lives and female life cycles when we discuss the [Goddess Archetypes.](#)

4. Incorporating Yoga into Your Journey

I'm sure you've heard that many clinical trials and studies have demonstrated the benefits of yoga for women in perimenopause (see all my references and links at the back if you want to look into this further.) In one randomized controlled trial, yoga was found to reduce the severity of hot flashes, improve quality of life, and decrease anxiety in women going through menopause. Another study found that a yoga intervention improved sleep, anxiety, and quality of life in perimenopausal women with insomnia. A review of several studies together, also indicated that yoga may be an effective non-pharmacological therapy for reducing menopausal symptoms, including those hot flashes, night sweats and mood disturbances. All of this shows (as if we need more evidence,) that yoga is not just fluff and is widely respected by the medical and scientific communities, and something we should most definitely be doing.

In addition to symptom relief, yoga has also been shown to have positive effects on cardiovascular health in menopausal women. A study found that a 12-week yoga programme improved arterial compliance and decreased arterial stiffness in postmenopausal women.

Overall, there is a ton of verified evidence to support the fact that yoga is an invaluable tool for managing the physical and psychological symptoms of perimenopause with its emphasis on breathwork, mindfulness and physical movement.

Whether you're just starting out with yoga or you are years into your yoga journey, it is important to find a style and teacher that resonates with you and is good for you at this life stage. I'm recommending that you seek out a local YogaPause teacher or join my online programme. It's always a good idea to start with a beginner class if you're new to yoga or one that caters to your newbie status, but make sure it's a practice that is serving your body as it is now.

How to Develop a Yoga Practice that Works for You and Your Body

Here, we'll explore the key components of your yoga practice and lifestyle that can help you achieve optimal health after forty.

First off, listen to your body. Your body may now be more sensitive to certain poses or movements, so it's important to be mindful of any discomfort or pain that you may experience. Always trust your instincts and avoid pushing yourself too hard.

It's important to remember that the most important aspect of your yoga practice is not the poses that you do, but how you do them. Focus on breathing deeply and mindfully and allow your body to find stillness and peace through each movement. Join the movement with the breath: For every inhale, an upward or outward movement. For every exhale, a downward or inward movement.

It is also super important to find a teacher or community that you feel comfortable with and that can support you during your yoga journey. Consider joining a class or workshop that specifically caters to women during perimenopause or working with a private teacher who can guide you through a personalised practice.

The YogaPause Sadhana

The YogaBellies Sadhana refers to those aspects of your yoga practice that make it effective in making your life better: The things that make yoga different from Zumba or Spin and more than just an exercise. I based The Sadhana around what I believe to be the five most important elements of any feminine yoga practice: Sense, Breathe, Move, Sleep and Circle. I'll explain what this means and how this relates to your menopause yoga journey.

Sense: Grounding and Embodiment

"Embodiment" means mindfully focusing on your body and being connected to your senses. It's also called interception in neuroscience. And when we're grounded, we're experiencing our mind, body, and breath all in the same place and at the same time. Sounds trippy, right?

Now, "grounding" can also mean "earthing," which is when you place your body in direct contact with the earth. In yoga, "grounding" often refers to feeling your body in contact with the earth, your yoga mat or other support, like a chair, to help you gain a sense of embodiment.

So, at the beginning of a YogaPause class, we take time to 'sense:' To be mindful and connected to our senses. To become aware of what's going on inside our body; how we feel right now and also what's going on in the external world around us. This can be particularly powerful as we move through life transitions like menopause, when it's often hard to accept the changes and discomforts we're experiencing.

To help you connect with your body and to initiate 'sense' at the beginning of your yoga practice, try this short exercise:

I like to begin this practice standing in Mountain pose or Tadasana at the top of my mat, but you can just as easily do this sitting in easy pose or lying down. Close your eyes and begin.

Take a few deep breaths, inhaling through your nose and exhaling through your mouth. As you exhale, imagine releasing any tension or stress from your body. Repeat this for a few breaths until you feel more relaxed.

Begin to bring your attention to your breath. Notice the sensation of the air moving in and out of your body. Observe how your chest and belly expand and contract with each inhale and exhale. Allow yourself to fully experience each breath, from the moment it enters your nose or mouth to the moment it leaves your body.

Now, bring your attention to your physical body. Start at the top of your head and slowly scan down through your body, noticing any sensations or areas of tension. Be curious and non-judgmental about what you feel. You might notice areas of warmth or coolness, tightness, or relaxation, tingling or numbness. As you become aware of each sensation, simply observe it without judgement or the need to change it.

If you notice any areas of tension or discomfort, you can direct your breath to that area, allowing it to soften and release. Imagine that with each exhale, you're letting go of any tension or discomfort, allowing it to dissolve into the space around you.

Now, you can turn your attention to the external world around you. Notice any sounds, smells, or other sensations in your environment. Tune into the larger universe. You might hear birds singing, the hum of traffic, or the sound of your own breath. You might smell the scent of flowers or feel the warmth of the sun on your skin. Allow yourself to become fully present in this moment, connected to both your internal and external experiences.

If you find your mind wandering, simply notice that it has wandered and bring your attention back to your breath or your physical sensations. Remember that it's normal for your mind to wander during meditation, and it doesn't mean that you're doing anything wrong.

Finally, take a few more deep breaths and slowly bring your attention back to your physical body. Wiggle your fingers and toes, and when you're ready, gently open your eyes. Take a moment to notice how you feel, both physically and mentally. You should now feel grounded and connected to yourself and the world around you and ready to begin your practice.

Breathe: Yogic Breathing

Yogic breathing techniques or pranayama have been used for centuries as a way to calm the mind, rejuvenate the body, and improve your health. They involve conscious control of the breath, which can have a profound impact on both body and mind for women at every life stage which is why it's such an important part of our practice. During menopause, breathing techniques can help reduce stress, the incidence of depression, and tension, and all sorts of common symptoms.

One of the main benefits of yogic breathing is that it increases self-awareness and centring. This is exactly what we need before we begin to move into our physical yoga practice. We should continue to connect the breath with the movements, creating a moving meditation as we continue our yoga practice. It's easy to feel overwhelmed and disconnected from yourself but by focusing on the breath, we can become more present in the moment and connect with what's really going on in our body and mind.

Pranayama also helps increase our focus and concentration. Practising yogic breathing can improve menopause brain fog, allowing us to think with a bit more clarity, and to feel more in control of the unstoppable changes.

Menopause sleep related issues and fatigue can make it a challenge just to stay awake during the day. Enter, Pranayama. Yoga breathing increases energy levels and helps you stay engaged in your day-to-day activities. It's also a great stress-reduction tool, as it activates the parasympathetic nervous system so that we can harness the body's relaxation response. It also increases the production of endorphins, which are natural mood enhancers that can help alleviate depression and promote that sense of positivity I keep pushing at you!

The Breath is an essential element of your YogaPause practice and not to be ignored. You'll find simple yogic breathing practices throughout the book for many of the menopausal symptoms you may come across. Try them out and see what feels right for you.

Move: Hit the Mat

Move is our Asana (physical posture) practice or what happens on the yoga mat. This is the mindful use of specifically chosen female-centric yoga postures to help you de-stress; tone-up and balance all aspects of your life.

A physical asana practice is an essential tool and by practising regularly, we are 'moving' which can alleviate a ton of physical symptoms and help us to feel more empowered and in control. Whether you are new to yoga or have been practising for years, incorporating a physical asana practice into your wellness routine is so powerful for overcoming the less pleasant aspects of perimenopause.

Sleep: And Relax...

'Sleep' is where we learn to relax deeply and completely, often during Savasana (the bit where you get to sleep) at the end of class. We also combine Yoga Nidra and self-hypnosis to induce the deepest levels of relaxation. These practices are all focused on releasing stress, and you can try out a combination of these tools to see which best suits your needs.

Savasana (or corpse pose) is typically practised at the end of a yoga practice, where you lie on your back with your arms and legs relaxed. This is all about surrendering and letting go, which can be incredibly helpful for relieving anxiety.

Yoga Nidra is a form of guided meditation that involves deep relaxation and visualisation. This practice can be especially helpful for women experiencing insomnia or difficulty sleeping. You can train your body and mind to relax deeply, which can help you fall asleep more easily and more importantly, stay asleep throughout the night.

Self-hypnosis involves inducing a state of deep relaxation and then making positive suggestions to your subconscious mind. This practice can be particularly helpful for women experiencing hot flashes, as self-hypnosis can help reduce the frequency and intensity. Additionally, self-hypnosis can be great to alleviate anxiety and increase feelings of well-being and self-empowerment.

Circle: Sisterhood

I believe that one of the most important and often overlooked aspects of practising yoga, is the sense of community that it can provide. This is something you get in a feminine yoga class, that you just won't find at the gym, where everyone runs out in the middle of Savasana. Yoga has the power to bring women together in a safe and supportive space, where we can share our experiences, offer each other support and encouragement, and find solace in the fact that we're not alone in what we're going through. Whether it's through attending a regular yoga class, joining a women's circle, or simply connecting with other women who are going through the same life stage, building a network of like-minded females can be incredibly empowering and healing.

In the yoga tradition, this sense of community is known as "Sangha." Sangha is the idea that we are all interconnected and that we need each other in order to thrive. This is especially true during times of transition and challenge, like menopause. By coming together, we can create a sense of belonging and shared experience that can help us navigate the unknown. There is nothing more reassuring than a sister telling you, "me too!"

One of the beautiful things about practising yoga in an all-female community, is that it allows us to let go of our individual struggles and connect with something larger than ourselves. This sense of connection can be incredibly healing, and it can help us find meaning and purpose. It can also help us feel seen and validated. We can share our stories, our struggles, and our victories with other women who truly understand what we're going through. This can help us to feel less isolated.

I encourage every woman to seek out community. Whether it's in person or simply connecting with other women online, finding a supportive community can make all the difference to your journey. By sharing our experiences and supporting each other, we can create a sense of connection and belonging that can help us find real meaning in our life again.

5. Yoga to Help Tackle 'Fun' Perimenopause Challenges

Let's explore our modifications a little further here. I want you to start thinking about what you're doing off the yoga mat too and what kinds of lifestyle modifications you can make to help you manage perimenopause challenges.

Insomnia and Sleep Disturbances

Insomnia is defined as difficulty falling asleep or staying asleep, and it is an absurdly common complaint among women during perimenopause. There are several reasons why insomnia often gets worse at this stage, including those pesky hormonal fluctuations and the related stress, as well as changes in our sleep patterns.

Fluctuating oestrogen levels disrupt the natural sleep-wake cycle and this leads to problems sleeping. Oestrogen helps regulate the circadian rhythm, which is the internal body clock that regulates our sleep-wake cycle, so when this randomly goes up and down, so is our ability to sleep soundly.

Stress is another factor that contributes to sleep related issues. Possibly being at the peak of our career, family responsibilities, grown-up kids that won't leave home, and alarming changes in our bodies: All of this stress can interfere with our natural sleep-wake cycle and worsen insomnia.

We will often experience more vivid dreams, night sweats, and frequent waking throughout menopause. Fortunately, there are several yoga practices that can help you get to sleep and stay asleep (whoop!)

Yoga Sequence for Insomnia

This is a really simple yoga sequence that will help with all kinds of sleep issues. Whether it's trouble getting to sleep; mid-night or premature waking; nightmares or night sweats, these postures will help you relax and release before bedtime.

Sukkhasana (Easy Pose): Sit cross-legged on the mat with your hands resting on your knees. Close your eyes and take a few deep breaths. This pose helps to centre the mind and reduce anxiety, which can often be the cause of insomnia.

Balasana (Child's Pose): Come onto your hands and knees, then sit back onto your heels and stretch your arms forward. Rest your forehead on the mat. Child's pose helps to calm the nervous system and relieve tension in the body too.

Supta Baddha Konasana (Reclining Bound Angle Pose): Lie on your back and bring the soles of your feet together, allowing your knees to fall open to the sides. Place your hands on your belly or out to the sides. Bound angle pose helps to relieve stress and promote relaxation. It's also a lovely hip-opener, and we tend to store a lot of emotional tension in this area.

Viparitta Kirani (Legs-Up-The-Wall Pose): Sit with your side next to a wall, then swing your legs up onto the wall as you lie back. Place your hands on your belly or out to the sides. This personal favourite helps calm racing thoughts and monkey mind (I used to sleep like this when I was pregnant!)

Uttanasana (Standing Forward Fold): Stand with your feet hip-width apart, then fold forward over your legs, letting your head hang heavy. This pose is fantastic to release tension in the back and shoulders, which often contribute to insomnia.

Adho Mukkha Svanasana (Downward-Facing Dog Pose): Come onto your hands and knees, then lift your hips up and back to form an upside-down V shape. This little puppy helps to stretch the hamstrings and relieve tension in the back and neck.

Ardha Matsyendrasana (Half Lord of the Fishes Pose): Sit with your legs straight out in front of you, then bend your right knee and cross your right foot over your left thigh. Twist your torso to the right, placing your left hand on your right knee and your right hand behind you. Repeat on the other side. This Asana helps to stimulate digestion and promote relaxation.

Savasana (Corpse Pose): Lie on your back with your arms and legs extended, palms facing up. Close your eyes and relax your whole body. I'm sure you know that Savasana helps you relax and sink into a beautiful, deep sleep.

Nadi Shodhana: Calming Breath for Insomnia

While there is no one-size-fits-all solution for insomnia, yoga breathing (pranayama) is great for helping you improve sleep quality. One specific pranayama practice that I love is called Nadi Shodhana, balancing breath or "alternate nostril breathing."

The slow, rhythmic nature of the practice helps you to relax, making it easier to fall and stay asleep. Also, by breathing deeply and evenly, it improves the flow of oxygen around the body, helping us relax even further. Incorporating Nadi Shodhana into your bedtime routine is a simple but really powerful tool for managing sleep issues. You can even do it in bed, making it nice and accessible, no special equipment needed. I've provided a basic version of the practice for you to try.

How To Do It:

To do Nadi Shodhana, find a comfortable seated position with a straight spine. Hold your right thumb over your right nostril and breathe in deeply through your left nostril. At the peak of the inhale, close off the left nostril with your ring finger and release your thumb from the right nostril, exhaling deeply. Next, inhale through the right nostril, close it off with your thumb, and exhale through the left. Repeat this process, alternating nostrils with each inhale and exhale, for several breaths.

Meditation for Peaceful Sleep

If you don't intend to go straight to sleep, you can try a short meditation to help clear your mind before settling down for the night:

Find a comfortable seated position, either cross-legged or on a chair. Close your eyes and take a few deep breaths. Imagine that you are lying on a soft, fluffy cloud. Feel the support of the cloud beneath you and let yourself sink into its softness. Notice the sensation of your breath moving in and out of your body. Let your mind be still, and simply observe your breath. If any thoughts or distractions arise, simply acknowledge them, and let them pass, like clouds drifting across the sky. Take a few more deep breaths, then slowly open your eyes, and come back to the present moment.

Hot Flashes

These can be uncomfortable, disruptive, and HOT, but there is also a lot of evidence to suggest that yoga can help. Yoga has a positive impact on the nervous system and hormone levels, which reduces the frequency and intensity of your hot flashes.

In addition, certain yoga postures, such as forward bends, child's pose, and savasana, can help regulate blood flow, which can provide some relief. Pranayama and mindfulness can also help regulate the nervous system, decreasing the impact of hot flashes. Improved sleep quality can help to reduce hot flashes even more, so all of those lovely insomnia practices come into play here too...

Here is a sequence that can be especially helpful for managing hot flashes during perimenopause.

Yoga Sequence for Hot Flashes

This sequence is designed to help regulate your body's temperature, calm your mind, and allow you release any stress or anxiety. By practising this sequence regularly, you may find that you're better equipped to cope with hot flashes and just feel more balanced and centred overall. Remember to listen to your body and take breaks during your practice when you need to, and always consult with your healthcare provider before starting any new exercise routine. Let's begin:

Sukkhasana (Easy Pose): Sit in a comfortable cross-legged position with your hands resting on your knees. Close your eyes and take a few deep breaths. Engaging in deep, diaphragmatic breathing in this pose activates the parasympathetic nervous system, responsible for the "rest and digest" response. Stress is a major trigger for hot flashes; by calming the nervous system, you mitigate the stress hormones that exacerbate hot flashes.

Bhujangasana (Cobra Pose): Lie on your stomach, with your hands under your shoulders and elbows close to your body. Inhale and lift your chest off the ground, keeping your elbows bent. Exhale and lower back down. Repeat for a few rounds. Cobra helps to stimulate the adrenal glands. These glands produce a variety of hormones, including cortisol and some sex hormones. Proper adrenal function can help in hormone regulation, mitigating hot flashes.

Supta Baddha Konasana (Reclining Bound Angle Pose): Lie on your back with the soles of your feet together, allowing your knees to fall open. Place your hands on your belly and breathe deeply into your belly, feeling it rise and fall with each breath. The open position of the hips and the focused deep breathing again stimulate the parasympathetic nervous system. This reduces the secretion of stress hormones, which can disrupt the body's temperature regulation mechanism and trigger hot flashes.

Viparitta Kirani (Legs Up the Wall Pose): Sit with your right hip against the wall, swing your legs up the wall and lie down on your back. Keep your arms by your sides, palms facing up. Elevating the legs promotes better blood flow to the pelvic area and heart. Improved circulation helps in better hormone distribution and can relieve the severity and frequency of hot flashes.

Surya Namaskara A (Sun Salutation A): Perform a few rounds of sun salutation, linking your breath with movement. This sequence helps to energise the body and increases overall circulation and oxygenates the body. Good blood flow ensures that hormones are well-distributed throughout the body, contributing to overall hormonal balance, which can help reduce hot flashes. If you've don't know Sun Salutation A, here is a break down:

Tadasana (Mountain Pose): Stand at the front of your mat with your feet hip-distance apart, palms facing forward. Inhale, and stretch your arms up overhead, palms together.

Uttanasana (Forward Fold): Exhale and fold forward from the hips, bringing your hands to the mat beside your feet. If you're not able to touch the mat, you can bend your knees slightly.

Ardha Uttanasana (Half Forward Fold): Inhale and lengthen your spine, bringing your hands to your shins or thighs.

Chaturanga Dandasana (Low Plank): Exhale and step back into plank pose. Lower down halfway, keeping your elbows close to your body.

Urdhva Mukkha Svanasana (Upward-Facing Dog): Inhale and roll over your toes, lifting your chest and pushing into your hands.

Adho Mukkha Svanasana (Downward-Facing Dog): Exhale and lift your hips up and back, forming an inverted V-shape with your body.

Ardha Uttanasana (Half Forward Fold): Inhale and step your right foot forward between your hands, coming into a lunge. Lift your chest and lengthen your spine.

Uttanasana (Forward Fold): Exhale and step your left foot forward to meet your right foot, folding forward over your legs.

Tadasana (Mountain Pose): Inhale and roll up to standing, reaching your arms overhead.

Repeat the sequence, this time stepping the left foot forward in step 7. You can repeat the sequence as many times as you'd like, linking each movement with your breath.

Savasana (Corpse Pose): Lie on your back with your arms by your sides and palms facing up. Close your eyes and focus on your breath, allowing your body to relax completely. In this pose, the body enters a state of deep relaxation and releases accumulated tension. The calming effect on the central nervous system can reduce the release of stress hormones, making you less prone to hot flashes.

Remember to keep your movements fluid and your breath steady. You can modify the sequence as needed, such as lowering your knees in Chaturanga Dandasana or taking a break in Child's Pose between rounds. Sun Salutation A is a great way to start your yoga practice or warm up your body for other postures.

In addition to these postures, it is important to cultivate that positive, pro-ageing mindset. You can work on this by practising gratitude, mindfulness, and yogic stress-management techniques, which we'll explore a little further on. Keeping a gratitude journal, engaging in daily meditation or deep breathing exercises, and finding healthy ways to cope with stress can all help promote a healthy mindset. If your head isn't in the right place, poor health is sure to follow.

Meditation To Ease Irritability Created By Hot Flashes:

As you lie in savasana, bring your attention to your breath. Notice the rise and fall of your belly with each inhale and exhale. Imagine a cool breeze flowing through your body, soothing any hot flashes. Repeat the following affirmations silently to yourself:

> *I am at peace with my body.*
>
> *My body is strong and healthy.*
>
> *I am calm and relaxed.*

Stay in savasana for as long as you like, enjoying the peace and stillness of the moment. When you are ready, gently bring yourself back to a seated position and take a few deep breaths before ending your practice.

Sitali Pranayama: Breath Practice for Hot Flashes

A yogic breathing practice or pranayama that is really helpful for hot flashes, is Sitali Pranayama, or "cooling breath." The act of breathing in cool air through the mouth can help bring down your body temperature and this can reduce the intensity of your hot flashes. Also, taking control of the breath alone, can help you feel less anxious and irritable. Deep breathing helps to increase the flow of oxygen around your body, and this is going to help to reduce the physical discomfort of hot flashes as well.

To do Sitali, find a comfortable seated position with a straight spine. Roll your tongue into a tube shape and stick it out of your mouth or purse your lips and breathe in slowly through your mouth, imagining that you are breathing in cool air. Hold the breath for a few moments, then exhale slowly through your nose. Repeat this process for several breaths, focusing on the sensation of coolness as you inhale.

Incorporating Sitali into your daily routine, or even just when you feel a hot flash coming on, can really help make hot flashes a bit more manageable. It's a simple but very powerful practice that can be done anywhere. However, it's important to listen to your body and only practice pranayama in a comfortable, relaxed manner. If you have any medical concerns, always consult with a healthcare professional before starting a new practice.

Menopausal Mood Madness

Once again, hormonal fluctuations are causing chaos in our bodies. Fluctuating oestrogen levels are one of the main causes of mood swings in menopause. The hormonal peaks and toughs impact the production of neurotransmitters, like serotonin, which regulates our mood. This results in off the scale, never seen before menopause mood swings, also known as 'the rage.'

In addition to temperamental hormones, stress and changes to your sleep patterns can also contribute to these mood swings. Vivid dreams, night sweats, and frequent waking, can disrupt the body's natural sleep-wake cycle, making mood swings even more dramatic.

Yoga To the Rescue (Again.) We've known mood swings since we got our very first period but here they are again, full force and punching! This yoga sequence includes poses that help with relaxation, balance your hormones, and reduce stress. By incorporating these postures into your practice, you can find a sense of balance during this transition.

Sukkhasana (Easy Pose): Begin by sitting in a comfortable cross-legged position with your hands resting on your knees. Close your eyes and take a few deep breaths, focusing on the inhale and exhale. Sukkhasana helps to calm the mind and reduce stress.

Bhujangasana (Cobra Pose): From a prone position on your stomach, place your hands under your shoulders and lift your chest off the ground, keeping your elbows close to your sides. This gentle backbend helps to stimulate the adrenal glands, which can be beneficial in balancing hormones.

Adho Mukkha Svanasana (Downward-Facing Dog Pose): From a tabletop position, lift your hips up and back, straightening your legs and forming an inverted V-shape with your body. Dog pose is perfect to relieve

Yoga to Help Tackle 'Fun' Perimenopause Challenges

stress and anxiety and can also help to regulate hormone levels.

Balasana (Child's Pose): From Downward-Facing Dog, bring your knees to the mat and sit your hips back onto your heels. Stretch your arms out in front of you, allowing your forehead to rest on the mat. This pose helps to release tension and relax.

Viparitta Kirani (Legs Up the Wall Pose): Lie on your back with your hips close to a wall and extend your legs up the wall. This pose is a great choice to help calm the nervous system and reduce stress, which can be helpful in managing mood swings.

Usttrasana (Camel Pose): Kneel on the mat with your knees hip-width apart and place your hands on your lower back. Slowly begin to arch your back and reach your hands towards your heels, keeping your neck long. Camel pose helps to open the chest and heart area and improve mood.

Savasana (Corpse Pose): Lie flat on your back with your arms and legs extended. Allow your body to fully relax and release any tension. This pose is a deep relaxation and is a relaxing reward at the end of your practice.

Each of these poses is helpful in managing perimenopause mood swings by reducing stress, balancing hormones, and calming the mind. Bhujangasana, Usttrasana, and Viparitta Kirani are especially beneficial for hormonal balance, while

Balasana and Savasana are great for relaxation and stress relief. Remember to listen to your body and modify the poses for your own level of flexibility and comfort.

Affirmations For Emotional Balance:

After your yoga sequence, find a comfortable seated position and close your eyes. Take a few deep breaths, then repeat the following affirmations to yourself:

I am calm and centred.

I am in control of my emotions.

I am at peace with myself and my surroundings.

Allow these positive affirmations to sink in and feel their calming effects on your mind and body. Stay here for as long as you like before gently opening your eyes and moving on with your day.

Brahmarri Breathing for Calming Mood Swings

Brahmarri Pranayama or "Humming Bee Breath" helps to activate the parasympathetic nervous system, which is responsible for the relaxation response in your body. This, in turn, reduces stress and anxiety, and helps you feel deeply relaxed. It helps to release any tension that you may subconsciously be holding in your body.

The humming sound produced during Brahmarri Pranayama has a vibration effect on your brain and body. This vibration stimulates the release of hormones like serotonin, which is associated with mood regulation, and oxytocin, which helps calm those spiking hormones even more. Win-Win!

Brahmarri Pranayama can be done at any time of the day, but it is recommended to practise it in the morning or evening for best results. Regular practice is going to help alleviate the severity and frequency of your mood swings, and just make you feel a whole lot more chilled.

To practise Brahmarri Pranayama:

- Find a comfortable seated position with your back straight and your eyes closed.
- Bring your awareness to your breath, taking a few deep inhales and exhales.
- With your lips gently closed, inhale deeply through your nose.
- As you exhale, make a humming sound like a bee, with your mouth closed and your teeth slightly separated.
- Continue to hum as you exhale, feeling the vibration of the sound throughout your body.

- Take a few more deep breaths with the humming sound on each exhale.

- After a few rounds of humming, release the sound and sit quietly, noticing any sensations or changes in your mood or energy.

Brain Fog

If you're experiencing brain fog, you're not alone. Many women report feeling forgetful, unfocused, and mentally cloudy during this time which can be both frustrating and concerning. Walking into a room and literally forgetting why you are there, can feel like you're losing your mind. But the good news is that there are things you can do to help manage this obnoxious symptom, including incorporating certain yoga and meditation practices into your routine.

First, let's talk about why menopause can cause brain fog. Oestrogen plays a key role in cognitive function, this includes your memory and attention span. So as those oestrogen levels dip, we start to experience things like forgetfulness, difficulty concentrating, and mental fatigue.

So, how can yoga and meditation help?

Stress can exacerbate brain fog and make it harder to focus and think clearly. Yoga and meditation both reduce stress, which in turn improves our cognitive function. Certain postures, like inversions (even simple ones like legs-up-the-wall pose,) can improve circulation to the brain, which can help support your brain health too. As you know, yoga has been shown to elevate mood and reduce anxiety, which results in less brain fog. Cultivating mindfulness and being present in the moment can help improve your focus and attention and reduce any mental clutter and distractions. An integration of all of these tools can positively impact the severity of menopause brain fog.

There are tons of studies showing why yoga is so important for women's cognitive stability as they get older. One study in 2017 published in the journal Menopause found that a 12-week yoga intervention improved cognitive function in postmenopausal women. The study included 49 women between the ages of 45 and 65 who were experiencing menopause-related cognitive decline. Participants were randomly assigned to either a yoga intervention or a control group. The yoga intervention consisted of 12 weeks of twice-weekly 60-minute yoga classes. At the end of the 12-week intervention, the yoga group showed significant improvements in cognitive function compared to the control group. This is one of many examples.

Here is a short yoga sequence to help improve cognitive function in perimenopause:

Sukkhasana (Easy Pose): Begin in a seated position with your legs crossed and your hands resting on your knees. Close your eyes and take a few deep breaths, focusing on the sensation of the breath moving in and out of your body. Sukkhasana is a gentle pose that can help to calm the mind and reduce anxiety.

Balasana (Child's Pose): From Sukkhasana, move into Balasana by bringing your forehead to the floor and reaching your arms forward. Allow your hips to sink back towards your heels and relax into the pose. Balasana is a restorative pose that can help to relieve tension in the neck, shoulders, and back.

Adho Mukkha Svanasana (Downward-Facing Dog): From Balasana, come onto your hands and knees and lift your hips up and back into Adho Mukkha Svanasana. Press your hands and feet firmly into the ground and lengthen through your spine. Downward-Facing Dog is a strengthening pose that can help to improve circulation towards the brain and increase energy levels.

Virabhadrasana II (Warrior II): Step your right foot forward and come into Warrior II by bending your right knee and extending your arms out to the sides. Turn your left foot slightly inwards and ground down through both feet. Warrior II is a powerful pose that can help to build strength and confidence.

Trikkonasana (Triangle Pose): From Warrior II, straighten your right leg and reach your right hand down towards the ground or a block. Extend your left arm up towards the ceiling and gaze up towards your left hand. Trikonasana is a pose that can help to improve balance and flexibility.

Ardha Chandrasana (Half Moon Pose): From Trikonasana, come into Half Moon Pose by placing your right hand on a block or the ground and lifting your left leg up towards the ceiling. Reach your left arm up towards the sky and gaze up towards your left hand. Ardha Chandrasana is a challenging pose that can help to improve focus and concentration.

Sethu Bandha Sarvangasana (Bridge Pose): Lie on your back with your knees bent and your feet flat on the ground. Press down through your feet and lift your hips up towards the ceiling. Interlace your hands underneath your body and roll onto your shoulders. Bridge is a gentle backbend that can help to relieve stress and tension.

Savasana (Corpse Pose): Finish your practice by coming into Savasana. Lie on your back with your arms and legs extended, allowing your body to completely relax. Close your eyes and focus on the sensation of the breath moving in and out of your body. Savasana is a restorative asana that can help reduce stress and anxiety.

You can finish your practice with this clarity meditation:

This meditation can help focus and concentration and lift those fluffy brain clouds. Begin by visualising a tranquil scene and focusing on a single object, you can begin to calm your mind and reduce stress and anxiety. Practising this meditation regularly can help you feel more grounded and centred, and to find more clarity in your thoughts.

Find a quiet place where you can sit comfortably for a few minutes without being disturbed. You can sit on the floor, on a cushion, or in a chair.

Close your eyes and take a few deep breaths, focusing on the sensation of the breath moving in and out of your body.

Bring your attention to the present moment and allow any thoughts or worries to drift away. Focus on the sensation of your breath moving in and out of your body.

Begin to visualise a peaceful and tranquil scene in your mind's eye. This can be any place that makes you feel calm and relaxed, such as a beach, a forest, or a mountain top.

Imagine yourself walking through this peaceful scene, taking in the sights, sounds, and smells around you. Feel the sun on your skin, the wind in your hair, and the ground beneath your feet.

As you walk, begin to focus on a single object in your surroundings, such as a flower or a tree. Allow your attention to be fully absorbed by this object, noticing every detail and texture.

If your mind begins to wander, gently bring your attention back to the object and continue to focus on it. Allow yourself to fully immerse in the present moment, letting go of any worries or distractions.

Take a few more deep breaths and bring your attention back to your body. Wiggle your toes and fingers, and slowly open your eyes.

Joint Pain

Fluctuating hormones can also impact the health of your bones and joints, leading to joint pain. You may have noticed creaky knees or hips that you didn't have before or maybe it's a dull throbbing or pain around certain joints. In addition, ageing and decreased physical activity can contribute to this joint pain. The low-impact nature of yoga, combined with its focus on strengthening and stretching, is going to improve your health and integrity of your joints and reduce any discomfort.

This short sequence for joint pain focuses on increasing your flexibility and mobility, easing any pain and helping you find some relief from the related stress. It's suitable for all levels and can be practised at any time of the day. It's also going to improve your circulation and decrease inflammation.

Yoga for Joint Pain

Begin by sitting in a comfortable cross-legged position and take a few deep breaths. Then, move into a slow warm up, with some gentle joint mobilisation exercises such as wrist and ankle circles, shoulder and hip rotations, and neck stretches.

Cat-Cow (Marjaryasana-Bitilasana): Come onto your hands and knees with your wrists directly under your shoulders and your knees directly under your hips. As you inhale, arch your back and lift your head and tailbone towards the ceiling (Cow Pose). As you exhale, round your spine and bring your chin to your chest (Cat Pose). Repeat this movement for 5-10 breaths.

Cat-Cow helps to warm up the spine, increase flexibility and mobility in the back, hips, and shoulders, and improve circulation to the joints.

Downward-Facing Dog (Adho Mukkha Svanasana): From hands and knees, press your hands and feet into the ground and lift your hips up and back, coming into an inverted V-shape. Keep your hands shoulder-width apart, and your feet hip-width apart. Hold for 5-10 breaths.

Downward-Facing Dog helps to stretch and strengthen the entire body, including the shoulders, hamstrings, calves, and ankles. It also improves circulation and reduces inflammation in the joints.

Warrior II (Virabhadrasana II): Stand at the front of your mat and step your left foot back about 3-4 feet. Turn your left foot out 90 degrees and your right foot in slightly. Bend your right knee and square your hips towards the front of your mat. Reach your arms out to the sides, keeping them at shoulder height. Hold for 5-10 breaths and repeat on the other side.

Warrior II strengthens the legs, improves hip flexibility, and stretches the groin and inner thighs. It also helps to improve balance and stability.

Tree Pose (Vrrkasana): Stand with your feet hip-width apart and bring your hands to your heart centre. Shift your weight onto your left foot and place your right foot on the inside of your left thigh. Press your foot and thigh together and bring your hands above your head. Hold for 5-10 breaths and repeat on the other side.

Tree Pose improves balance, strengthens the ankles and legs, and stretches the hips and inner thighs. It also helps to calm the mind and reduce stress and anxiety.

Seated Forward Fold (Paschimottanasana): Sit on your mat with your legs straight in front of you. Inhale and reach your arms up overhead. Exhale and fold forward, reaching towards your feet. Hold for 5-10 breaths.

Seated Forward Fold stretches the hamstrings, hips, and lower back. It also helps to improve digestion and reduce stress and anxiety.

Body Scan Meditation for Dealing with Pain and Discomfort

A really simple yogic meditation practice that can help you manage pain and joint discomfort is a basic Body Scan Meditation. You can try this one from my YogaPauseTV YouTube channel. This practice involves lying down or sitting in a comfortable position and focusing the mind on the sensations of the body, helping you relax and feel more connected to what's happening inside your body.

A Body Scan Meditation is perfect for when you're dealing with physical discomfort or emotional turbulence, by focusing on the sensations of the body. It can help to identify, release and reduce any pain related to tension. It increases your awareness of the feelings and physical sensations in your body, and it can be especially helpful when trying to identify and address the source of your pain.

Start by closing your eyes and taking a few deep breaths, allowing yourself to settle into the moment. Then, begin to focus your awareness on your body, starting with your feet and working your way up to the crown of your head. As you focus on each part of your body, take a moment to notice any *sensations* or sensations of discomfort.

Repeat to yourself:

> *I am strong and capable of overcoming any challenge.*
>
> *My body is healing and becoming more flexible and mobile.*
>
> *I am grateful for the benefits that yoga brings to my mind and body.*

As you scan your body, imagine that each part is becoming more and more relaxed and at peace. Take deep breaths and focus your awareness on the sensations of your breath moving in and out of your body. If you find your mind wandering, simply bring your focus back to your breath and the sensations of your body.

Menorrhagia (Heavy Periods)

As a result of our bodies producing less oestrogen and progesterone, our periods can become more irregular and heavier (or lighter!), and this varies greatly among women and can be impacted by other factors too.

But why would periods get heavier, you might ask. Surely if my menstrual cycle is coming to an end, they would get lighter?

Well, as our hormone levels fluctuate, the lining of our uterus can become thicker than usual, which can cause heavier bleeding when we do have a period. Additionally, as we get older, our blood vessels can become more fragile, which can also contribute to heavier bleeding too.

Menorrhagia (or heavy periods) are defined as menstrual bleeding that lasts more than seven days or requires changing tampons or pads every two hours or less. It can be a symptom of various conditions, including hormonal imbalances, uterine fibroids, or endometriosis, and it's important to speak with a healthcare provider if you experience heavy periods so that you are aware of all of the options and get the support that you need. They may or may not be related to perimenopause, but it's always best to check it out, especially if you are in pain.

Yoga for Heavy Menstrual Flow

So, if your periods have become heavier as well as random AF, this is the sequence for you. As someone who suffered from debilitating periods (think migraine; cramps that had me bed-bound and nausea,) I have personally effectively used this sequence many times.

Balasana (Child's Pose): Begin by kneeling on your mat with your big toes touching and your knees hip-width apart. As you exhale, slowly lower your torso down to rest your forehead on the mat, stretching your arms out in front of you. Rest your arms alongside your body, palms facing up. Hold this pose for at least 30 seconds, breathing deeply and allowing yourself to relax.

This gentle forward fold helps to relieve stress and anxiety, which can contribute to heavier periods. It also helps to stretch the hips, thighs, and ankles.

Viparitta Kirani (Legs-Up-the-Wall Pose): Sit on the floor with your right hip close to a wall. Slowly lie back onto the floor with your legs extended up the wall. Your hips should be close to the wall, and your legs should be straight up the wall. Rest your arms alongside your body, palms facing up. Hold this pose for at least 5 minutes, breathing deeply and allowing yourself to relax.

This pose helps to calm the nervous system and further reduce anxiety. It also helps to increase blood flow to the pelvic area, which can be helpful for menorrhagia.

Supta Baddha Konasana (Reclining Bound Angle Pose): Begin by sitting on your mat with your legs extended in front of you. Bend your knees and bring the soles of your feet together, letting your knees drop out to the sides. Slowly lower your torso down to rest on the mat, keeping your feet together and knees out to the sides. Rest your arms alongside your body, palms facing up. Hold this pose for at least 30 seconds, breathing deeply and allowing yourself to relax.

This posture helps to open the hips and relieve tension in the pelvic area. It also helps to calm your monkey mind and help you de-stress.

Usttrasana (Camel Pose): Begin by kneeling on your mat with your knees hip-width apart. Place your hands on your hips and inhale, lifting your chest up. As you exhale, slowly lean back, bringing your hands down to your heels. Keep your hips forward and your thighs vertical. Hold this pose for at least 30 seconds, breathing deeply and allowing yourself to relax.

This gentle backbend helps to relieve tension in the chest and upper back, which can contribute to menorrhagia too. It also helps to improve posture and increases your energy levels.

Ardha Matsyendrasana (Half Lord of the Fishes Pose): Begin by sitting on your mat with your legs extended in front of you. Bend your right knee and place your right foot on the outside of your left knee. Place your left hand on your right knee, and your right hand behind your right hip. Inhale, lifting your chest up. Exhale, twisting to the right, looking over your right shoulder. Hold this pose for at least 30 seconds, breathing deeply and allowing yourself to relax. Repeat on the other side.

This twist helps to stimulate the digestive system and improve circulation to the pelvic area. It also helps to relieve any tension in the spine and improve flexibility.

Savasana (Corpse Pose): Lie on your back on your mat with your legs extended and your arms at your sides. Close your eyes and allow your body to fully relax. Breathe deeply and let go of any tension or stress in your body.

Hold this pose for at least 5 minutes, breathing deeply and allowing yourself to relax.

This allows the body and mind to completely relax and to let go of any tension or stress. It also helps to promote a sense of calm.

Remember to always listen to your body and modify the postures as needed and don't forget those probs. Heat and ice packs can be particularly helpful for cramps too and you can add those into a restorative practice. This sequence can be done anytime, but it is especially helpful when your periods are painful or heavier than usual.

A Meditation To Get You Through Heavy Periods:

Menorrhagia can be debilitating, I know, and I've been there. Try this meditation to help you settle your mind and manage any pain and to help balance the associated hormonal fluctuations.

Find a comfortable seated position or lie down in Savasana. Close your eyes and take a deep breath in through your nose, filling your lungs with fresh air. Hold for a moment, then exhale slowly through your mouth, letting go of any tension or stress. Take a few more deep breaths like this, allowing your body and mind to relax more and more with each exhale.

As you breathe, visualise a beautiful, calming blue light filling your body and soothing any discomfort or pain caused by menorrhagia. Allow this blue light to spread throughout your body, from the top of your head down to your toes, bringing peace and tranquillity to every part of you.

Stay here for as long as you like, allowing yourself to fully relax and let go of any worries or concerns. When you're ready to come out of the meditation, take a deep breath in and slowly exhale. Gently open your eyes, feeling refreshed and rejuvenated.

Osteopenia and Bone Health

Decreased bone density is a common issue for women during and after menopause. This decrease in bone density can be due (again) to hormonal fluctuations and changes in lifestyle, which can also increase the risk of osteoporosis and other bone-related conditions. As if we didn't have enough to worry about...

Yoga (obviously) is great for improving bone health and reducing the risk of osteoporosis. The weight-bearing nature of many yoga postures, combined with the focus on strengthening and stretching, can massively improve your bone density and overall joint health. This is one of the many reasons why yoga is so popular as women get older. Here are some postures to focus on if improving bone density is a current focus or concern for you.

Yoga Sequence for Osteopenia

If increasing bone density is of specific concern for you right now or you just want to get ahead of the bone health game, here is a quick and easy yoga sequence for Osteopenia:

Tadasana (Mountain Pose): Stand with your feet hip-width apart, rooting down through your feet and lifting your spine. Reach your arms overhead and interlace your fingers, palms facing upward. This posture strengthens the legs and spine, which can help prevent bone loss in the legs and lower back.

Uttanasana (Standing Forward Bend): From Tadasana, hinge forward at the hips and fold over your legs, letting your hands rest on the ground or a block. Uttanasana stretches the hamstrings and back muscles while also promoting blood flow to the head, which can help reduce stress and tension that can contribute to osteopenia.

Adho Mukkha Svanasana (Downward-Facing Dog): Start on your hands and knees, with your wrists under your shoulders and your knees under your hips. Curl your toes under and lift your hips up and back, straightening your arms and legs. This pose strengthens the arms, shoulders, and legs while also increasing blood flow to the head and reducing stress.

Virabhadrasana II (Warrior II): Step your right foot forward and bend your right knee, keeping your left foot planted and your left leg straight. Reach your arms out to the sides, parallel to the ground. The Warrior postures strengthen the legs and hips, which can help prevent bone loss in these areas.

Trikonasana (Triangle Pose): From Warrior II, straighten your right leg and reach your right hand forward, then place it on a block or the ground. Reach your left arm up toward the ceiling. Triangle stretches the legs and side body while also strengthening the core, which can help support the spine and prevent bone loss in the torso.

Sethu Bandha Sarvangasana (Bridge Pose): Lie on your back with your knees bent and your feet flat on the ground. Press down through your feet and lift your hips up toward the ceiling, interlacing your fingers underneath your back. Practising Bridge pose strengthens the legs, hips, and back while also promoting bone density in the spine.

Viparitta Kirani (Legs-Up-The-Wall Pose): Sit with your left side against a wall, then swing your legs up the wall and lie back with your head and shoulders on the floor. This posture promotes blood flow to the legs and helps reduce swelling and inflammation in the feet and ankles, which can be common in people with osteopenia.

Savasana (Corpse Pose): Lie on your back with your arms at your sides, palms facing up. Close your eyes and take several deep breaths, relaxing your entire body. This posture allows your body to rest and rejuvenate, which can help reduce stress and promote an overall sense of wellbeing.

A Meditation for Strong, Healthy Bones

Osteopenia and Osteoporosis can be a big concern as we get older and there is literally, no exercise better than yoga to help prevent and ease these conditions. If you are currently suffering from decreased bone density you may be in pain or struggling with the idea that this is happening to you. This meditation will help you focus on staying strong on the inside and out.

Begin by finding a comfortable seated position, either on a cushion or a chair with your feet firmly on the ground. Close your eyes and bring your awareness to your breath, taking deep inhales and exhales.

As you breathe, imagine a warm, healing light surrounding you, filling you up from the top of your head to the tips of your toes. Visualise this light bringing strength and resilience to your bones and muscles, helping to support and protect your body.

Now bring your awareness to any areas of tension or discomfort in your body. Breathe into these areas, allowing the warmth of your breath to soften and release any tension or pain.

As you continue to breathe deeply, bring your attention to your mind. Notice any negative thoughts or worries that may be weighing you down. Visualise these thoughts as dark clouds, and imagine a gentle breeze blowing them away, leaving behind clear, blue skies.

As you let go of negative thoughts and worries, focus instead on feelings of gratitude and positivity. Think about all the things in your life that bring you joy and happiness and allow these feelings to fill you up from within.

Finally, take a moment to set an intention for yourself. Whether it's to stay committed to a regular exercise routine, eat a balanced diet, or practice self-care, set a clear intention that will help you stay strong and healthy in body and mind.

Take a deep breath in, and exhale slowly, allowing yourself to fully embody your intention. When you're ready, gently open your eyes, feeling renewed and empowered to face whatever challenges may come your way.

No time to meditate? Try repeating these positive affirmations when symptoms flare up or you're feeling low:

My body is strong and healthy.

I am capable of healing myself.

I trust my body to take care of me.

I am grateful for the strength and resilience of my bones.

I am at peace with my body and my journey through perimenopause.

Other Ways You Can Improve Bone Density

As our bodies start producing the oestrogen essential for maintaining nice, strong bones, there are several other ways you can help increase your bone density. Try to incorporate some if not all of these into your routine:

- Weight-Bearing Exercise: ramp up activities like walking, jogging, dancing, or resistance training help to increase bone density. These are a good addition to your yoga practice. These types of exercise work by putting stress on your bones which stimulates new bone growth. Try to do at least 30 minutes of weight-bearing exercise every single day, whether that's yoga or a simple walk in the park. Another great idea is to add in some hand weights to your yoga practice. I've included a YogaPause Strong sequence to try further on in the book.

- Calcium-Rich Diet: This is essential for maintaining strong bones. Foods like dairy products, leafy green vegetables, nuts, and seeds are all excellent sources of calcium. Aim to get at least 1000-1300 mg of calcium every day if you can.

- Vitamin D: Vitamin D helps the body to absorb calcium, so you must ensure you are getting enough of it. Foods like fatty fish, egg yolks, and mushrooms are all good sources of vitamin D. If you are not getting enough vitamin D from your diet, consider taking a supplement.

- Avoid Smoking and Limit Alcohol: Both can have a really negative impact on bone density. If you smoke, try to quit, and if you enjoy a little vino, limit your intake to no more than one drink a day. I know this can be a tough one ladies, especially if you've been using alcohol for 'stress relief.' I do love a Cosmo, but facts are facts and alcohol is also a depressant, so start looking at healthier stress relieving alternatives that actually work.

- Get Enough Sleep: Essential for good health, and especially important for maintaining strong bones. Aim to get at least 7-8 hours of sleep every night.

If this is a major concern for you right now, it's important that you talk to your doctor about what steps you can take to maintain healthy bones too.

Menopausal Middle and Weight Gain

Hormonal changes have a significant impact on your body composition and metabolism. This can lead to weight gain at a noticeably increased rate and possibly in specific problem areas that were never previously a problem.

One of the main reasons for menopause weight gain, is the decrease in oestrogen which regulates our weight by controlling the distribution of fat in the body. When oestrogen declines, we tend to accumulate more fat around our midsection, often referred to as the "menopausal middle." The cherry on top of this excess belly fat, is that it's particularly dangerous and is associated with an increased risk of heart disease, diabetes, and other health problems too.

Our metabolism also slows down as we get older. Our bodies require fewer calories to maintain our weight, which means that we need to eat less and exercise more to maintain the same healthy weight. This means that bingeing on Big Mac's at the weekend and fitting comfortably into size 8 jeans, is probably a thing of the past. Many of us find it difficult to reduce our calorie intake and increase our physical activity levels, which can make weight loss after 40 a real challenge.

When I turned 40, it felt as if I put on a stone overnight and it was *all* around the belly area, where it had never been before (thighs had always been my personal fat magnet.) I'm not too worried about it though, as my focus now is on being strong and healthy as opposed to "skinny." Instead of trying to lose the fat I've turned it into muscle and I'm really happy with how I look and feel. I'd much rather be toned, active and happy than starving and stick thin.

Stress contributes to weight gain as well and what is more stressful than unwelcome changes to your body and mind? Emotional overeating and sleep disruption related to stress can further impact our metabolism, causing us to gain even more weight: Stress on stress!

Weight gain at this point in life is a concern for most women. However, it's not impossible to maintain a healthy weight. By implementing a mindful approach to eating, proper nutrition, moving and practising yoga regularly, managing stress in healthy ways, getting enough sleep, and considering hormone replacement therapy... It can be done. It's just a little more challenging!

If weight-gain is something that concerns you, mix up your practice with a more dynamic and flowing yoga. Dive into the chapter on eating mindfully and I also recommend that you try Intermittent fasting.

Yoga to Help Tackle 'Fun' Perimenopause Challenges

Try this yoga sequence to improve your circulation, strengthen your muscles, and increase your energy levels. It will also help to reduce stress and improve digestion, which can be important factors in managing weight gain. Remember you cannot 'spot tone' with any exercise so focus on a whole body practice, that tones and helps you lose or maintain weight all over.

Sun Salutations (Surya Namaskar). Stand at the front of your mat and go through the flow that includes poses like Mountain Pose, Forward Fold, and Plank. It's a great way to get your blood pumping and wake up the body, setting a positive tone for the rest of your practice.

Mountain Pose (Tadasana), stand tall with your feet hip-width apart and your arms by your sides. Inhale, raising your arms overhead. This basic but powerful pose improves posture, strengthens your legs, and gives a burst of energy.

Forward Fold (Uttanasana) by exhaling and folding from the hips, reaching your hands towards the mat. Feel the stretch in your hamstrings and the release in your lower back. It's like a sigh of relief for your spine and a tranquilliser for a stressed mind.

From here, transition into **Plank Pose (Phalakkasana).** Step your feet back and align your body in a straight line from your head to your heels. Hold your core tight. This pose is a full-body toner, making you strong and stable, much like a human plank of wood.

Cobra Pose (Bhujangasana). With your legs extended behind you, press the tops of your feet into the mat as you lift your upper body. This move gives your back muscles a good workout and encourages spinal flexibility, which can be a real mood-lifter.

Step one foot between your hands and rise into **Warrior I (Virabhadrasana I).** Your front knee is bent while the back leg is straight, arms reaching skywards. This is a power pose that fortifies your legs, hips, and back, and makes you feel like, well, a warrior.

Warrior II (Virabhadrasana II). Your front knee stays bent, but now both arms extend out in line with your shoulders, and you gaze over your front hand. This posture is a hip-opener and circulation booster that helps you stay grounded.

Chair Pose (Uttkatasana). From standing, bend your knees as if you're sitting back in a chair, extending your arms overhead. Feel the burn in your legs, and maybe even a little in your soul. It's all worth it for those toned thighs and improved posture.

Bridge Pose (Sethu Bandha Sarvangasana). Come onto your back and lift your hips towards the ceiling while pressing your feet into the mat. This pose is an antidote to hours of sitting—it stretches your chest, neck, and spine and gives your legs and glutes a good workout.

End with **Camel Pose (Ustrasana).** Kneel on the mat, then arch your back to reach for your heels. This one opens up the whole front line of the body, from your chest to your abdomen. It's almost like your body is saying 'thank you' as you stretch and strengthen.

Body Positive Meditation

This meditation will allow you to indulge in a little self-love and help cultivate positivity as your body changes. This is really important during a time when these changes might be difficult to accept. By repeating meaningful, positive affirmations and visualizing a warm and loving light, this meditation can help to boost your self-esteem and reduce any negative self-talk. Focus on cultivating a loving, positive relationship with your body.

Begin by finding a quiet and comfortable place where you can sit or lie down for a few minutes without being disturbed. Take a few deep breaths, inhaling through your nose and exhaling through your mouth.

Close your eyes and bring your attention to your body. Notice any areas of tension or discomfort and allow yourself to fully accept and acknowledge these feelings without judgement.

Repeat the following affirmations to yourself, either out loud or in your mind:

I am beautiful and worthy, just as I am.

My body is strong and capable of amazing things.

I trust my body and its natural processes.

I honour and respect my body, treating it with kindness and compassion.

I release any negative thoughts or feelings about my body and embrace self-love and positivity.

Visualize yourself surrounded by a warm and loving light, filling you up with positive energy and self-love. Allow this light to permeate your entire being, washing away any negativity or self-doubt.

Focus on your breath, inhaling deeply and exhaling slowly. Imagine any tension or stress melting away with each exhale, leaving you feeling calm and centred.

Take a few more deep breaths, and when you're ready, slowly open your eyes.

6. An Extra Something: Incorporating Weights into Your Perimenopause Yoga Practice

Adding light weights to your yoga practice can bring a new level of intensity, help you build strength, tone your muscles and improve your bone density. Incorporating weights can also help you increase your metabolism. Using weights in your practice helps to increase resistance and further your efforts.

So, how can you incorporate weights into your yoga practice without hurting something?

There are a few different approaches you can take, like using hand weights, ankle weights or gloves or a weight vest. I'm a fan of hand and wrist weights. Whichever method you choose, it's important to start slowly and gradually increase the weight as you build your strength and confidence.

Start by using light hand weights during your sun salutations—0.5, 1 or 2 kg are perfect. Holding a weight in each hand as you move through each pose can help you engage your core, build upper body strength and improve your balance. Another option is to add weights to your Warrior poses, which can help you build strength in your legs, hips and glutes.

You know how important it is to listen to what your body needs, and yoga is not about no pain, no gain. If it hurts, you should stop. If you feel exhausted or experience discomfort, you may need to reduce the weight or take a break from using weights altogether.

Remember to focus on proper form. When performing Asana with weights, be mindful of your alignment and use your breath to maintain control and balance. It's important to engage your core and use the weights to help deepen your stretch, rather than relying on them for balance. Don't go crazy with big, heavy weights. Proper alignment, the right postures and small weights are much more effective.

It's also a good idea to start with basic yoga postures and gradually progress to more complex movements as you become more comfortable with the weights. Even if you're a yogini expert, you may start with a simple Warrior I pose and add a light dumbbell to each hand. As you become more comfortable, you can progress to more challenging postures like Triangle or Half Moon and slightly increase the weight.

Another great way to incorporate weights is to use them in a flowing sequence. This can help you to develop greater strength, flexibility and coordination while also improving your balance and mindfulness. You can try a simple flow like sun salutations, adding a lightweight to each hand, or try a more complex flow that incorporates multiple postures and movements.

By building and maintaining muscle mass, you can reduce the risk of injury, manage the worst symptoms of perimenopause, and achieve greater overall strength and flexibility. So why not give it a try?

Remember to always listen to your body and be mindful of your breath and alignment when performing any yoga postures, especially when using weights.

10 Yoga Postures You Can Try With Weights

Here are ten yoga postures that you can practice with weights and an explanation of how to do this and why.

Warrior III with Dumbbells: This one's not for the faint-hearted, but oh boy, does it pack a punch for your balance and lower body. Stand tall, feet hip-width apart, dumbbells in hand, arms overhead. Move your weight onto your left foot and slowly hinge forward, lifting your right leg and lowering your torso. Hold that air-surfing pose for 5-10 breaths. Switch sides.

Balancing Table to Downward Dog with Dumbbells: This dual pose is like a two-for-one deal: a stretch and a strengthener. Start on all fours, a dumbbell in your right hand. Extend that arm and your opposite leg out, forming a straight line. Take five breaths, and then jazz it up by lifting your hips into Downward Dog. Hold for another 5-10 breaths and give the other side some love.

Chair Pose with Dumbbells: You've done Chair Pose, but have you ever tried it with weights? Stand with feet hip-width, dumbbells in hand, arms up. Sit back into that imaginary chair. You'll not only feel the fire in your legs but get a lovely stretch across your upper body. Hold, breathe, release.

Tree Pose with Dumbbells: Tree Pose is like the yoga equivalent of a warm hug. Stand tall, then place your right foot on your left thigh or calf. Dumbbell in your right hand, raise it skyward. This move works on your balance and strength, making you feel like the goddess of multitasking. Switch after 5-10 breaths.

Cobra Pose with Dumbbells: Cobra Pose, but make it weighty. Lie face down, dumbbells in hand. Press up, lifting your upper torso off the mat. Hold and breathe, feeling those back muscles awaken. Hold for 5-10 breaths.

Warrior I with Dumbbells: Ready for another warrior pose? Of course you are. Dumbbells in hand, step back with your left foot and bend the right knee. Hoist those dumbbells up, making sure your arms know they're part of the action too. Hold the pose for 5-10 breaths, and then switch sides.

Triangle Pose with Dumbbells: Stretch and strengthen is the name of the game here. Start with feet apart, dumbbells in hands. Reach towards your right foot with your right hand and stretch your left arm to the heavens. Hold for 5-10 breaths, and switch.

Seated Cat-Curl with Dumbbells: Find yourself in Hero Pose, dumbbells in hand. Arch your back on an inhale, and round it as you exhale. Go through several breath cycles, really syncing movement and breath.

Plank Pose with Dumbbells: It's plank, but with an edge. Get into plank position with a dumbbell in each hand. Keep everything tight for 5-10 breaths and switch sides if you like.

Child's Pose with Dumbbells: Finish it off with a few minutes of relaxation in Child's Pose. Place your forehead on the mat, and slide your arms forward, dumbbells in hand. Hold and breathe for 5-10 breaths.

And that's your modern yogic adventure with a weighty twist. Remember, this is yoga, not the weightlifting Olympics. It's about blending strength and flexibility into one seamless flow.

7. Your Lovely Yoni (and it's a sad decline!)

Here, we're going to explore what nobody wants to talk about—Vaginal Atrophy or 'your vagina getting old.' We'll look at what the dreaded vaginal atrophy is, what causes it and what you can do to mitigate the worst of it.

Although you may have thought about getting older, you probably didn't spend sleepless nights worrying about your vagina getting older or what that actually means. Vaginal atrophy affects most women during the menopause journey, to a greater or lesser extent. Like every other problem in life over forty, it's caused by a decrease in oestrogen. This can lead to thinning, drying and inflammation of the vaginal walls, which can result in things like dryness, itching, burning and even pain during intercourse.

Although it inevitably comes to us all, some women suffer more severe symptoms. There are a few things that put you at higher risk of having more issues with VA:

- Smoking

- Hormonal birth control medications or devices like the patch or implant

- Synthetic hormones

- Low sex hormones (oestrogen, progesterone or testosterone)

- Autoimmunity

While vaginal atrophy can be uncomfortable and even painful, don't panic: There are lots of options available to manage it.

Natural Options for Vaginal Restoration

The good news? Vaginal atrophy is preventable and even somewhat reversible. New treatments and therapies are becoming available all the time, from lasers to

If you prefer a more natural approach to managing atrophy, you may want to start with these simple steps.

Dietary changes: Eating phytoestrogens can help increase your oestrogen levels naturally. Stock up on foods such as soy, flaxseeds and chickpeas are all rich in phytoestrogens. Focus on foods that support a healthy gastrointestinal tract and vaginal pH.

Probiotics: Take a Lactobacillus-Based Probiotic. Lactobacillus acidophilus is the best probiotic for establishing healthy vaginal balance. Two other strains researched for vaginal health are lactobacillus rhamnosus and lactobacillus reuteri.

Herbal remedies: There are many herbal remedies that help improve vaginal dryness and discomfort. Black cohosh and red clover are two herbs that are often used. I'll discuss Yoni Steaming and useful herb blends for this stage of life here too.

Lifestyle changes: Things like quitting smoking and engaging in regular movement and exercise, can also help a lot. You know that drinking plenty of water is essential for maintaining your general health, but it can also help with symptoms of vaginal atrophy. Staying hydrated helps keep your vaginal tissues happy, comfortable and moist and can reduce friction.

Yoni Yoga: I'm sure you've heard of them, but Kegel exercises involve contracting and relaxing the pelvic floor muscles. They can help strengthen your pelvic floor and improve blood flow to the area too.

A yogic twist on this is yoni yoga. You can do this with or without a yoni egg and you can fast forward a few pages to find out exactly what this is and how to do it. Like kegels, it involves contracting and holding the muscles in and around the vagina. The beautiful thing about yoni yoga, is that you can incorporate this into your daily yoga practice or make it a dedicated practice in itself.

Try Mula Bandha (The Root Lock/Loch): *Mula bandha* (the root loch) is a yogic practice that involves engaging the pelvic floor muscles. This is not a 'Kegel exercise', but on a physical level, Mula Bandha strengthens your pelvic floor and counteracts the gravitational pull on the bladder and reproductive organs. Mula Bandha is also believed to stimulate the endocrine and excretory systems, which can help to prevent low mood and depression.

Many styles of yoga recommend holding Mula Bandha throughout your yoga practice in order to keep the energy (prana) flowing in and up instead of down and out. The rationale is that this internal lift gives you more upward energy and helps ward off tiredness.

Quick Pelvic Girdle Anatomy 101: Let me explain a little about the pelvic girdle, just so that we're all on (literally) the same page. It's shaped like a bowl and is made up of three fused bones—the ilium, ischium and pubis. At the bottom of the pelvis, there's an opening called the pelvic outlet. The perineum, which is shaped like a diamond, is at the base of the opening. The coccyx or the base of the spine is located at the rear of the diamond while the front of the diamond is called the pubic symphysis or the joint between the two pubic bones. The two sit bones are located at the left and right corners of the diamond.

When it comes to Mula bandha, it's associated with the centre of the perineum. Some yoga texts suggest that you can apply light pressure below the area to stimulate contraction, for example, sitting on a rolled-up sock or a specially designed cushion. For women, the contraction of the Mula bandha is felt in the area surrounding the base of the cervix.

To practise Mula bandha, you can focus your attention on the back, front or middle of the perineum or multiple areas at the same time. The key is to learn to activate the perineum at its centre.

Yes, Mula Bandha is an ancient, spiritual and often complex practice, but fear not, I am here with a preliminary version for you to try.

- Find a comfortable seated position: You can sit cross-legged on the floor or sit on a chair with your feet firmly placed on the ground.

- Bring awareness to your perineum: The perineum is the area between the anus and the genitals. You can bring your attention to this area by simply focusing your mind on it.

- Contract your perineum muscles: Imagine that you're trying to hold in urine or gas. Contract the muscles in the perineum and pull them up towards your navel.

- Hold the contraction for a few seconds: Once you've contracted your perineum muscles, hold the contraction for a few seconds, then release it.

- Repeat the process: Practise this contraction and release process for a few minutes, taking short breaks in between if necessary.

Remember that Mula bandha can take time to master, and this is just a basic instruction on how to get started. It's important to be patient and not to get discouraged if you don't get it right away, especially if you feel disconnected from this area of your body generally. With consistent practice, you'll gradually build connection, strength and control. Additionally, it's always best to seek the guidance of a qualified yoga teacher if you're unsure about the technique or experience any discomfort while practising it or want to learn a bit more.

Avoid irritants: Products like perfumed soaps, lotions and douches can irritate vaginal tissues and exacerbate VA symptoms. Forget the foaming, strawberry feminine hygiene products. Avoid using these like the plague and opt for gentle, unscented, natural and organic products whenever possible.

Try natural and water-based lubricants during sex to reduce friction and improve comfort: Lubricants will not fix the underlying problem, but they will help you manage the symptoms. Natural lubricants work well, and they will not complicate the situation further. Examples of vaginal lubricants include things like Replens and Astroglide.

Moisturize. Similar to lubricants, vaginal moisturizers can also help relieve dryness and irritation. They're designed to be used on a regular basis to help maintain your vaginal happiness. Examples include Hyalo Gyn and Luvena, although there are a lot on the market so you may want to try a few and see what feels best for you.

Some essential oils that can help to moisturise the vaginal canal include rose, lavender, Cape chamomile, Roman chamomile, frankincense and sandalwood. Make sure to procure your essential oils from trusted sources. Then dilute them before mixing them with either olive oil, coconut oil or vitamin E oil. However, keep in mind that these oils are not safe to use with condoms.

Wear cotton underwear and avoid tight-fitting clothing to allow for better ventilation too. I have no affiliation whatsoever, but I highly recommend Calvin Klein undies if you haven't discovered them. I am also a big fan of my 'big pants', which are 100% cotton, come right up to my waist and come in a pack of 5 for two quid from Primark.

Laser therapy: This is a relatively new option that involves using a laser to stimulate collagen production in the vaginal tissues. The idea is that by increasing collagen production, you can improve vaginal elasticity and reduce dryness and discomfort.

One great thing about laser therapy is that it's minimally invasive and typically doesn't require any downtime. You'll likely need multiple treatments over the course of a few months, but the procedure itself is relatively quick and painless. Plus, many women report significant improvement in their symptoms after undergoing laser therapy. There are different types available for example, MonaLisa Touch appears to be the celebrity favourite, as well as FemTouch and FemiLift.

Of course, like any medical treatment, laser therapy may not be right for everyone. It's important to talk to your healthcare provider about your symptoms and individual needs and your health status before making any decisions. But if you're looking for a modern and effective treatment option for vaginal atrophy, laser therapy is definitely worth considering!

Vaginal atrophy happens, but there are so many options available to manage it. The main thing is to become aware of what's going on down there, not just around your period (or the lack of it.) Are you experiencing discomfort or itching? What feels like regular thrush, or an irritation could be VA. Whether you prefer medication, natural remedies or lifestyle changes, there are ways to alleviate these painful symptoms and prevent it from affecting your overall quality of life. Stay tuned for a few more of my favourite natural vulva self-care practices after we discuss meds.

Medication and Hormones

One of the most common treatments for vaginal atrophy is medication. Yep, it's time to talk HRT (hormone replacement therapy) There are several types of medication available to treat VA, let's have a look.

HRT is a treatment option that involves taking oestrogen or a combination of oestrogen and progesterone to replace the hormones that we lose during perimenopause and menopause. You're not adding in 'new' hormones, just replacing those ones that we've seen that we need for pretty much everything, but are now in rapid decline. HRT can help improve problems like dryness, itching, burning and pain during sex. Oestrogen creams, which are used topically on the vulva area, have also been shown to have fewer side effects than other forms of HRT and focus on relieving the symptoms only in this area.

So, what are the different HRT options available for managing vaginal atrophy?

Systemic HRT: Systemic HRT involves taking oestrogen or a combination of oestrogen and progesterone in pill, patch, gel or spray form. This type of HRT can help manage symptoms throughout the body, including hot flashes, mood swings and bone loss. Now, this is a super top-line overview of HRT, but I discuss this in a lot more detail in The YogaPause online programme, or you can get in touch with your favourite gynae for more information.

Local oestrogen therapy: This involves using oestrogen creams, tablets or rings that you place directly into the vagina or apply around the vulva area. This type of HRT is specifically designed to target vaginal atrophy symptoms and can help improve vaginal lubrication and comfort during sexual activity. Use Bioidentical Progesterone as progesterone plays a vital role in our reproductive health, as progesterone is declining.

Combination HRT: Combination HRT involves taking both oestrogen and progesterone to replace the hormones that we're losing during perimenopause. This type of HRT can help manage symptoms throughout the body (hot flashes, night sweats, etc.) and as well targeting your vaginal atrophy symptoms.

While HRT can be a really effective treatment option for vaginal atrophy, it is important to know that there are some risks and side effects associated with this treatment, so you should most definitely discuss the most up to date options with your healthcare provider.

Yoga for Your Vagina

Yoni Love: Yoni Yoga Sequence

I believe in giving my vagina a lot of love. Some of the practices I swear by include yoni yoga—with and without a yoni egg—and also vaginal or yoni steaming. I'll explain how these practices can help keep your vulva happy, including adapting your yoga practice and lifestyle for Yoni love. Let's explore some of the ways you can do this.

An easy one. Incorporate yoga poses that increase blood flow to the pelvis. Certain yoga poses can help increase blood flow to the pelvic region, which can help alleviate vaginal dryness and discomfort. A few of my favourite poses are below, but I've also included a couple of yoni yoga postures for you to try later.

- **Malasana** (garland pose): This involves squatting down with your feet and knees wide apart, allowing your pelvic floor muscles to stretch and relax.

- **Baddha Konasana** (bound angle pose): This pose involves sitting with the soles of your feet together and gently pressing your knees down towards the floor, creating a gentle stretch in the pelvic area.

- **Janu Sirsasana** (head-to-knee pose): This posture involves sitting with one leg extended and the other foot resting against the inner thigh. Gently fold forward over your extended leg, allowing your pelvic floor muscles to release.

Practising these poses can definitely help increase blood flow and reduce VA symptoms.

Try using props for support.

Using props like blankets, cushions, bolsters, and blocks for your yoga practice can give you a bit more support and comfort during poses that could aggravate the vulva area. For example, you could try using a blanket to sit on during seated poses to help reduce pressure on the pelvic region and take some pressure off, especially if you're experiencing pain down below. Heat packs can be a saviour too.

Yoni Love: A Yoni Yoga Sequence

Yoni yoga is a powerful practice that will increase blood flow to that special lady region, strengthen your pelvic floor muscles, help you to reconnect with your body and just relax! If you are currently suffering from vaginal atrophy or you want to get one step ahead, yoni yoga can be a great tool. This can be done with or without the use of a yoni egg (see further down for more on this.)

Here is a yoni yoga sequence that you can try (without an egg for now):

Bound Angle Pose (Baddha Konasana): Sit on a yoga mat with your legs extended in front of you. Bend your knees and bring the soles of your feet together, allowing your knees to drop out to the sides. Use your hands to gently press down on your thighs, encouraging your knees closer to the floor. Take a few deep breaths and then release. This pose improves hip flexibility and helps you focus.

Butterfly Pose (Supta Baddha Konasana): Lie on your back with your knees bent and the soles of your feet together. Allow your knees to drop out to the sides. Place your hands on your belly and take a few deep breaths, feeling the rise and fall of your abdomen.

Bridge Pose (Sethu Bandasana): Lie on your back with your knees bent and your feet flat on the floor. Press your feet and arms into the floor and lift your hips towards the ceiling. Hold for a few breaths and then release. This not only strengthens your glutes but also engages your core.

Goddess Pose (Uttkata Konasana): Stand with your feet wider than hip distance apart and turn your toes out to the sides. Bend your knees and lower your hips down towards the floor, keeping your spine straight. Place your hands on your thighs and take a few deep breaths. This pose is good for toning the lower body and helps you build stability.

Pelvic Tilts: Lie on your back with your knees bent and your feet flat on the floor. Inhale and lift your hips towards the ceiling. Exhale and release. Repeat several times, focusing on using your pelvic floor muscles to lift your hips. This subtle movement focuses on engaging your pelvic floor muscles.

Reclined Bound Angle Pose (Supta Baddha Konasana): Lie on your back with your knees bent and the soles of your feet together. Allow your knees to drop out to the sides. Place a pillow or blanket under your head for support. Close your eyes and take several deep breaths, allowing your body to relax completely.

As you practise this yoni yoga sequence, remember to focus on your breath and listen to your body. If any pose feels uncomfortable, feel free to modify or skip it.

Try this short meditation at the end of your yoni yoga practice:

Sit comfortably with your eyes closed, taking a deep breath in through your nose and exhaling out through your mouth.

As you continue to breathe deeply, bring your attention to your yoni area. Feel the warmth and energy that you have generated through your yoni yoga practice.

Visualise a bright white light surrounding your yoni and filling it with healing energy. Feel any tension or discomfort melting away.

Repeat the following affirmations to yourself silently or aloud:

I am strong and capable of facing any challenge.

I trust my body and its natural processes.

I am connected with and love and respect my Yoni.

I am at peace with myself and my experiences.

I am grateful for all that my body has given me.

I am open to receiving love and support from those around me.

Take a few more deep breaths, feeling a sense of calm and contentment wash over you.

When you're ready, gently open your eyes and take a moment to acknowledge the positive energy you've created within yourself.

Let's Talk Yoni Eggs

A Jade egg or yoni egg practice is the ancient Chinese art of using yoni eggs to literally heal the body from the inside out. This 5,000-year-old practice was once the closely guarded secret of the royal Chinese concubines, but it is now being rediscovered by women worldwide. I discovered that this awesome practice is said to not only tighten the pelvic floor and improve your sexual health, vitality and the intensity of your orgasms but also provides a myriad of other cracking benefits. Ancient texts promised benefits such as a natural facelift, longevity, curing incontinence, improved lubrication and decreased menstrual cramps. I can honestly say that through my practice over the past 10 years, I've experienced every one of these benefits.

I knew that this was something I had to bring to other women, so I created Yoni Love. I started to combine a gentle yoga practice with the use of my Jade Egg to create a complete spiritual and physical practice. Yoni Love is about being comfortable in your own body. We've been taught to be ashamed or embarrassed by our own reproductive organs and our physical and sensual needs as a woman. Not only can a yoni yoga practice help with this, but it's also a deeply healing practice. Women who have suffered traumatic childbirth or even sexual assault can truly heal by working through these emotions.

You can just wear your Jade Egg while you go about your daily business, or even wear it to bed, but I highly recommend you combine the practice with the gentle asana or Yoni Love sequence I've included. This allows you to fully engage all the internal muscles, so you get a gentle and therapeutic workout.

Not only is a regular practice great for vaginal health, but it is also great for your mental and emotional health. The practice of yoni yoga is a moving meditation: It helps calm and balance the mind and helps you reconnect with and appreciate your body.

It cures incontinence!

Inserting a Jade egg into the vagina strengthens your Mula bandha (root lock) and is also said to seal in your vital energy or Chi. On the most basic physical level, it tightens your pelvic floor, helps to resensitize the vaginal canal and stops you from peeing yourself: What's not to like here?

It contains vital life force or prana in the body.

On an energetic level, when the PC muscle and diaphragms become loose, life-force energy will leak out from the organs as they tend to stack upon each other. This can cause conditions such as prolapse as the organs drop all their weight to rest upon the perineum.

Using a Jade Egg in the vagina also stimulates the vaginal reflexology points relating to the liver, lungs, heart, spleen and kidneys allowing for even more benefits of this practice. When we practise Yoga Asanas while wearing the egg, as opposed to a static yoni egg practice, even more of these points are activated as you're moving around, enhancing the benefits even further.

It keeps you looking young and feeling vibrant!

One of my favourite books ever, *Vagina* by Naomi Wolf (a Yale graduate and former political advisor to Bill Clinton), mentions the direct connection of the vagina to the brain and even a direct correlation to a woman's confidence. This radiates in the face providing that secret glow. When these muscles are strengthened by Yoni Love, no energy is leaked from the root lock. This means we maintain this vitality which was said to result in a natural facelift which kept the royal concubines youthful.

It can regulate your menstrual cycle and help to alleviate PMS.

Yoni yoga can help to alleviate PMS and even hormonal imbalances in perimenopause. Healthy sexual organs mean decreased pain, cramping and even fewer PMS during your menstrual cycle, which is great as your cycle goes haywire! A regular yoni yoga practice can tone the internal vaginal canal and organs and help reduce a lot of heavy bleeding, cramping and fatigue.

It improves lubrication and vaginal elasticity.

The increased circulation using your yoni egg helps you lubricate naturally. This especially applies during and after menopause. Yoni yoga can also help return vaginal elasticity. For a physically and energetically healthy vagina, Jade eggs are most definitely the way to go: Tight, moist and happy vaginas all around.

It helps get your libido back, heightens sexual pleasure and can make you multiorgasmic.

A yoni egg practice awakens the vaginal tissue allowing you to experience deep vaginal orgasms. We're so used to things being carelessly 'shoved' into the vagina: Tampons, penises, fingers ... that the vagina can tense up, freeze, and numb over time. By showing our vaginas some gentle consideration and love, we can resensitize and invigorate those muscles again. If you've never experienced vaginal, G-spot, cervical or full-body orgasms (I hadn't), then these portals of pleasure will now become open to you.

Strengthening the pubococcygeus muscles, allows us to enjoy longer-lasting, more powerful and more intense orgasms. This was something I experienced after only using the yoni egg a handful of times. Not only that but you will be able to isolate the rings of muscles in the vaginal canal, enabling you to 'squeeze' your partner during intercourse, meaning your partner will feel the benefits too.

My advice to you: Purchase a Jade Egg as soon as possible. Find a qualified teacher and learn the range of gentle Yoni asanas to accompany your jade egg practice. Enjoy all of the benefits you didn't even know you could experience from yoga.

Here's how to choose and use a yoni egg:

Choose the right egg. Yoni eggs come in a variety of sizes and materials, so it's important to choose one that is comfortable and appropriate for your level of experience. If you're a beginner, start with a medium-sized egg made of a non-porous, easy-to-clean material like nephrite jade. You may see cheaper eggs in obsidian or rose quartz, but Nephrite Jade was chosen by the emperor's concubines for a reason: It's unbreakable, non-porous and rare. Invest wisely!

Clean and prepare the egg. Wash the egg thoroughly with warm water and mild soap, and then rinse it with hot water to sterilise it. You can also place the egg in boiling water for a few minutes to ensure it is fully sanitised.

Insert the egg. Lie down in a comfortable position and gently insert the egg into your vagina, with the larger end first. Never force it. Allow yourself to relax and allow your yoni to gently 'sip' the egg in. Hold the egg at the base of the vagina and breathe in and out using the muscles around the entrance to bring it inwards. A gentle nudge is allowed. Allow your pelvic floor muscles to hold the egg in place and relax and breathe deeply.

As with any new practice, it's important to start slowly and listen to your body. If you experience any discomfort or pain, stop immediately. Wearing a yoni egg should never hurt!

Practice yoni yoga. Once the egg is inserted, you can even try a yoni yoga practice. The poses and movements are similar to those practised in traditional yoga, but with a focus on engaging the pelvic floor muscles and working with the yoni egg.

Remove the egg. When you're finished with your yoni egg practice, gently remove the egg from your vagina and clean it again with warm water and mild soap. Store it in a safe and dry place until your next practice.

Try some of these poses when using your egg during yoni yoga:

Pelvic Tilts for Core & Pelvic Floor Awareness: Lie on your back, knees bent, feet flat. Inhale, lifting your hips towards the ceiling while engaging your pelvic floor muscles around your yoni egg. This helps improve pelvic floor strength and core stability. Exhale and lower your hips.

Squats for Lower Body & Pelvic Floor Strength: Stand with your feet hip-width apart, toes turned out. Lower into a squat, keeping your spine aligned. This posture enhances lower body strength and, thanks to your yoni egg, engages the pelvic floor. Hold briefly and rise back up.

Goddess Pose for Stability & Pelvic Floor Engagement: Feet wider than hips, toes out, lower your hips towards the ground, engaging your pelvic floor muscles to keep the yoni egg in place. This pose is great for pelvic floor strength and overall stability.

Warrior II (Virabhidrasana II) for Leg & Core Toning: Stand with your feet wide apart. Turn your right foot out and bend the right knee, extending arms parallel to the ground. The posture not only tones your legs but the engagement required to hold the yoni egg also works on your pelvic floor. Hold, then switch sides.

Triangle Pose (Utthita Trikonasana) for Core & Spinal Strength: From Warrior II, straighten the front leg and extend your torso over it, placing your hand on the shin or floor. The other arm reaches skyward. This engages the core and the back, and yes, your pelvic floor won't be left out if you're mindful of the yoni egg.

Boat Pose (Navasana) as a Core Intensifier: Sit down, bend your knees, and lift your legs into a V-shape, balancing on your sit bones. Extend your arms forward. This pose is all about the core, and engaging the pelvic floor will add an extra layer of stability.

Cat Curls (Bidalasana) for Back Flexibility & Core Engagement: On all fours, alternate between arching your back as you look up (cow) and rounding it as you look down (cat). This improves back flexibility and when you add a pelvic floor squeeze around the yoni egg, it's a bonus for your core as well.

Leg Raises for the Lower Back & Core: Lie on your back, legs straight. Raise one leg at a time while keeping the other on the floor. As you lift, engage your core and pelvic floor to maintain the position of the yoni egg. This is excellent for lower back and core strength.

Child's Pose (Balasana) for Relaxation & Deep Engagement: From all fours, lower your hips back to your heels and extend your arms forward. Although a restful pose, you can use this moment to focus deeply on engaging your pelvic floor around the yoni egg.

Yoni Egg Practice Meditation

If you're struggling to get comfortable with your yoni egg or having trouble relaxing enough to insert the egg, you could try reading this meditation while allowing the body to relax fully.

Sit or lie down in a comfortable position and take a few deep breaths. As you begin your yoni egg practice, focus your attention on your breath and the sensation of the egg in your yoni.

Visualise a warm, soothing light glowing in your pelvic area, bringing healing and comfort to your reproductive system. As you inhale, imagine this light growing brighter and more intense, filling your entire body with healing energy. As you exhale, release any tension or discomfort you may be holding in your yoni and pelvic area.

Repeat these affirmations to yourself:

I honour and appreciate my body, and the changes it's going through during this phase of life.

My yoni is strong, healthy, and capable of healing itself.

I am open and receptive to the wisdom and guidance of my body.

I trust in the natural processes of my body and the universe.

Visualise the yoni egg as a tool to amplify your intention for healing and self-love. Imagine the egg absorbing any negative energy or blockages in your yoni, and filling you with positive, healing energy.

Stay with this visualisation and these affirmations for as long as feels comfortable, allowing yourself to fully relax and let go. When you're ready, gently remove the yoni egg and take a few deep breaths before ending your practice.

Yoni Steaming

When I first heard about vaginal steaming, my initial reaction was 'What!?' However, as someone who has suffered from nausea, migraines, debilitating cramps and the wildest of wild PMS over the years, I was willing to try anything.

Yoni or vaginal steaming is the term used to describe steam treatments, not just to the vagina area, but the entire "yoni." You can listen to my podcast on it here.

The word 'yoni' is Sanskrit in origin and is the symbol of the Hindu divine mother, goddess Devi or Shakti. Ancient cultures believe that the womb and the yoni are the seats of all well-being and health in a woman and that we could remedy most ailments by coming back to the womb and realigning. This philosophy has been re-embraced in recent years with women moving back toward more traditional remedies to solve issues where modern medicine may have failed us.

Yoni steaming is so effective that it's practised across the world for centuries, and I found out that it has many names, including:

- In the West, it is known as a 'Vaginal Steam' or 'V Steam'.

- Mayans called it 'Bajo', which means low in Spanish and refers to the crouching position often taken to steam.

- In Korea, it is called 'Chai-Yok'. It's especially popular here, with chains of franchised 'v-steam' stores on every street corner. Many Korean women choose to steam daily!

In cultures worldwide and throughout history, yoni steaming has remained a well-respected ritual for supporting all aspects of women's general health and wellness—not just related to vaginal or womb health. Purported benefits range from the physical to the emotional and even the spiritual. Yoni steaming is an ancient and established remedy that has crossed borders and timelines and frankly, it frickin' rocks.

Why the hell should I steam my vagina?

This practice can help treat painful periods, dysmenorrhea, irregular menses, yeast infections, UTIs, perineal or vaginal tears, fibroids, etc; it can enhance fertility and can improve ovarian or vaginal cysts, scarring from C-sections, or even haemorrhoids. It can also assist in easing pain from painful intercourse, vaginal dryness caused by menopause or contraception, and much more. For me, it helped regulate irregular menses, heavy bleeding, and cramps that I suffered from after multiple miscarriages.

The specific herbs we choose in yoni steaming encourage the shedding of excess build-up in the uterine lining every month, and for women struggling with infertility, yoni steaming helps to nourish and tone the uterine lining. It helps to relax the cervix and the vaginal canal and in turn, increases cervical fluid and reduces dryness.

What can you expect after steaming?

Often, after you begin practising yoni steaming, you will notice your menstrual cycle may change. The practice will often expel a great deal of encrusted material from your womb. The chosen herbs will dislodge anything stuck in the uterine passage, including this old residue. Your menses may be unusually dark, heavy and thick for a couple of days, and the length of your period could extend or reduce, depending on the blend used. Ultimately, your next period should be much lighter, and life will become much more pleasant.

Want to try basic yoni steaming at home?

You will need the following:

- A slatted or modified bamboo, canvas or wood chair or stool to let the steam through. Alternatively, you can just use your toilet bowl.

- Two large natural cotton or wool blankets.

- A large stainless steel stock pot to hold and boil one gallon of water.

- A large Pyrex, ceramic bowl, or sitz bath to hold the steaming liquid (the liquid with the herbs).

- A cup of your dried herbs or premade yoni steam blend of choice or a one-quart mason jar filled with fresh herbs.

Choosing your herbs

Since experiencing the benefits of yoni steaming firsthand, I then went on to train professionally as a yoni steam facilitator. I strongly recommend you purchase some pre-blended herbs from a professional blender or make a basic "general" steam, as recommended below. However, if you are looking to remedy specific ailments, it is best to work with a yoni steam facilitator to make sure you get the correct schedule and blends or buy a pre-made Perimenopause blend like this one. You can use one to five steaming herbs or vaginal herbs for your steam:

- Traditional herbs: yarrow, plantain, damiana, chamomile, rosemary, marigold, basil and oregano

- Great herbs for perimenopause: Lady's Mantle, Yarrow, Red Raspberry Leaf, Damiana, Motherwort, Marshmallow Root & Shatavari Root

How to do it

- Put the blanket near the chair or toilet bowl.

- If using a chair or stool, find a comfortable area for your chair.

- Boil the herbs in water for about 15 to 30 minutes.

- If using a chair or stool, pour the steaming liquid into a pot or bowl. Place under the chair or stool.

- If using the toilet bowl, pour the steaming liquid into a large bowl. Put the bowl into the toilet bowl.

Note: the easiest, least expensive and best item to use for your yoni steaming is a sitz bath. Pour one to two cups of the steaming liquid into the sitz bath.

- Let the steaming liquid sit for about 30 to 60 seconds to let it cool slightly. Test the steam. The genitals are very sensitive to heat, so you need hot steam—not scalding. Hover the inside of your forearm over the steam to test if the heat is comfortable.

- Remove your clothes from the waist down, including your underwear. You need to be half-naked for this.

- Sit on the chair or toilet bowl. Cover the entire lower half of your body with the blanket; cover all the way to the ground, making a tent, to keep the steam inside.

- Steam for 20 to 30 minutes. You can read a book, listen to music or write while steaming.

- After steaming, rest in a warm room, without air conditioning, without open windows and free of drafts, for at least 20 minutes.

- Dress in clothes that will keep you warm and protect you from sudden temperature changes or cold drafts for 24 hours.

How often should I steam?

Treatment schedules will vary (see your yoni steam professional!), but for general wellness, yoni steams one week before your menstruation are great for preventative care. For endometriosis, fibroids, pelvic pain, prolapse and cysts, do yoni steaming two to four times weekly. After a miscarriage or D&C procedure, wait at least three weeks and make sure you have no infection before yoni steaming. After giving birth, wait for about six to eight weeks and make sure you are no longer bleeding and have no infection before steaming.

Important reminders

Don't steam during menstruation or pregnancy, if you have open wounds or infections, if you have an IUD or if you have symptoms of moist or damp heat in the vagina, pelvis or colon, which could mean a herpes outbreak, bacterial infection, yeast infection or vaginal infection.

Choose the right time in your menstrual cycle. Yoni steaming is typically done during the second half of the menstrual cycle, after ovulation and before menstruation begins. It is not recommended during menstruation, as it can interfere with the natural flow of blood and lead to potential infection.

Use a safe and sturdy steaming station. Choose a steaming stool or chair that is specifically designed for yoni steaming or use a regular chair with a hole cut in the centre. Make sure the stool or chair is sturdy and stable to prevent accidents.

Don't steam for too long. Yoni steaming should be done for no more than 30 minutes at a time and only once per week. Over-steaming can cause burns, dryness and other vaginal irritations.

Practise good hygiene. Make sure to thoroughly clean your yoni and the surrounding area before and after steaming and avoid using any harsh soaps or other products that could irritate.

Listen to your body. If you experience any discomfort or pain during yoni steaming, stop immediately and consult with a healthcare provider.

Overall, yoni steaming can be a helpful tool for addressing vaginal atrophy and promoting overall vaginal health during perimenopause. It's relaxing, cleansing, invigorating and therapeutic all at once, and it has truly changed my menstrual cycle for the better.

Yoni Steaming Meditation

Here's a meditation that you can read while practising yoni steaming. This may help you relax and embrace the practice and to set your intentions for your Yoni steaming session:

Close your eyes and take a deep breath in through your nose, and exhale through your mouth with a soft sigh.

Now, bring your awareness to your yoni area, where the steam is gently rising up to heal and nourish your body. Visualise this warm, soothing steam permeating every cell of your being, bringing balance and harmony to your reproductive system.

As you inhale, repeat the following affirmations silently to yourself:

My yoni is a sacred space, deserving of love and care.

I am grateful for this opportunity to nurture my body and spirit.

I trust in my body's natural ability to heal and balance itself.

I release any negative thoughts or emotions, and welcome in peace and joy.

As you exhale, feel any tension or stress melting away from your body, replaced by a sense of calm and well-being.

Continue to repeat these affirmations with each inhale and allow yourself to fully surrender to the healing power of the steam.

When you are ready to finish, take a deep breath in, and exhale with a soft sigh. Gently open your eyes and take a moment to feel the warmth and lightness in your body.

Remember to give yourself the love and care that you deserve, and trust in the natural process of your body as you navigate through perimenopause.

8. PMS: Is It Getting Out of Hand?

Around 85 percent of menstruating women suffer from one or more of the symptoms of PMS every month, and this goes up in perimenopause. You know when it hits. That week before your period when you are overcome by crazy, unable to control your mood swings, and basic logic becomes a vague memory.

You may have other symptoms like breakouts of teen spots, sore boobs, bloating, joint or muscle pain, random food cravings, mood swings, or suffer from severe irritability and anxiety. Let us not forget the irrational thinking, backaches, cramps and depression. Diarrhoea, headaches, migraines and insomnia are also some of the pains that we may endure monthly.

Why does PMS get worse during perimenopause? Well, of course it has to do with hormone fluctuations. During our menstrual cycle, our hormone levels naturally fluctuate, which can cause physical and emotional symptoms. However, during perimenopause, these fluctuations can become more severe and unpredictable, leading to more intense PMS symptoms.

One of the most common PMS symptoms that can get worse during perimenopause are mood swings.

Hormonal fluctuations can cause anxiety, irritability and even depression or rage. You may find that changes in mood become more severe during perimenopause as the hormonal shifts are greater.

Another symptom that can get worse is bloating and as our hormones rocket up and down, we can experience increased water retention and bloating. This can be particularly frustrating as the bloating can be more severe and longer lasting. Yoga is GREAT for this one too.

Menstrual irregularities can also contribute to worsening PMS. As our menstrual cycles start to become irregular, it makes it even harder to predict when these symptoms will occur which can be frustrating and make it harder for us to manage.

So, what can we do to manage worsening PMS symptoms? Yoga.

How so?

Yoga helps by balancing the endocrine system, and gentle stretching when practising yoga releases any increased muscle tension generated by our internal hormonal stresses. Yoga regulates our breathing and improves circulation around the body, as well as helping with any menstruation-related digestive issues, like constipation or diarrhoea.

Many of us that already have an existing yoga practice avoid practising in the days leading up to our period, simply because we're exhausted or feeling low. However, there are some postures and practices that can be really beneficial as we approach the start of our menstrual cycle. Don't be afraid to make your practice comforting and restorative, because that is exactly what you need at this time.

Yoga for PMS

Try practising the following postures in order, as a sequence or individually, to help ease the symptoms of PMS.

Pigeon pose or *Eka Pada Rajakapotasana* is a great posture for releasing tension in the hips and groin and allowing yourself to completely chill. Pigeon pose can help relieve tightness and restore flexibility.

Place your hands on your lower back and gently arch your back. You should feel a nice stretch in the front of your left hip, but if this variation is painful, lean forward, placing your hands on the floor in front of you. Hold for five or more breaths, and then repeat this pose on the other side.

***Natarajasana* or Dancer's pose** requires a significant amount of flexibility in the hip flexors and spine, as well as an unwavering sense of balance. Benefits include reducing menstrual discomfort and PMS symptoms.

Begin in Tadasana and stretch the right arm forward and keep it parallel to the ground. Bend the left knee toward the back and hold the left big toe with the left hand. Engage the knees and press the left foot into the left hand to lift it up and to the back. Keep the balance for 10 seconds then release the grip of the left foot and lower the arms. Repeat the posture on the other side.

Beginners can practise this pose by placing the front hand on a wall for balance. They will still feel a fantastic stretch and feel all the emotional benefits, too.

Usttrasana or **Camel pose** helps to stimulate the thyroid gland in the centre of the neck to balance metabolism and affects the entire endocrine system.

Come up onto the knees. Reach your hands back one at a time to grasp your heels, and then bring your hips forward so that they are directly over the knees. Allow the head to come back, opening your throat and chest.

If this is too much of a stretch to reach all the way back to the feet, just gently kneel and take the hands to the hips. Look up toward the third eye (between the eyebrows) and bend gently backwards as much as is comfortable. Take the shoulders back and down and open the chest as you bend backwards from the hips.

Dhanurasana or **Bow** pose is a great back bending pose, which will help to stimulate the reproductive organs and helps to balance the levels of progesterone and oestrogen in the body. It stimulates both the back and front of the body, especially the lumbar and pelvic regions and helps relieve depression. Combat cramps and upset stomachs with a backbend like this pose, which gets the spinal fluid moving and relieves compression in the vertebrae.

Lie on your belly with your hands by your side, with your palms up. On the exhale, bend your knees and bring your feet toward the buttocks. Reach back and take hold of the ankles. The knees should only be a hip distance apart, if possible. Inhale, lift the heels away from the buttocks and lift your thighs from the floor. Your head and chest will follow and lift off the floor. Keep your back muscles soft.

Continue to lift, press the shoulder blades together and open the chest. Draw the shoulders away from the ears. Gaze forward while breathing more into the back. Breathe here for about five seconds, release with an exhale and repeat once or twice, comfortably.

If grabbing the feet is too much of a strain, you can use a strap around the front of the feet and reach back and grab the strap. Remember you don't have to come all the way up, either; for many people, just grabbing the ankles and raising the chest is enough of a stretch.

Uttitha Parsvakonasana or Extended Side Angle pose strengthens and stretches the legs and knees and opens the groin and waist region. While stimulating the abdominal organs, this posture can also provide us with an influx of energy at times when we are feeling lethargic and fatigued.

Stand with feet facing forward, about four feet apart. Raise the arms parallel to the floor and reach them out to the sides, with the palms down, stretching with the fingertips. Turn your left foot in slightly to the right (about 45 degrees) and your right foot out to the right (about 90 degrees). Align the heels and turn the right thigh outward, so that the kneecap is above the ankle. Bend the front knee, anchoring with the heel of the back foot.

Take the shoulders back and down and extend the left arm up toward the sky, with the left palm facing toward your head and then reach the arm up and over. Lengthen from the heel to the tips of the fingers. Turn your head to look at your fingertips.

Hold for five breaths and then change sides and reverse the feet. Then come up and return to *Tadasana*.

The postures should be held for five breaths each, but if you feel able, you can repeat the flow as many times as you wish up to 10 times. If the posture is practised on the left and right, then hold for five breaths on each side.

Please note that this sequence is to be practised 'before bleeding begins'. When menstruation begins, we should abstain from all practice for the first three days or focus on meditation and yogic breathing, 'pranayama'.

Meditation For PMS:

Finish this practice with a short meditation and some positive affirmations. Sit or lie down in a comfortable position, close your eyes, and take a few deep breaths. Then, repeat the following affirmations to yourself:

I trust my body and my intuition.

I acknowledge any pain or discomfort in my body and let it go.

I see my thoughts passing through my mind like clouds, I am not attached to my thoughts.

I am strong and capable of handling any challenges that come my way.

I am deserving of love and compassion, especially during difficult times.

I release any negative thoughts and feelings and embrace a sense of peace and calm.

Allow yourself to rest in this state of calm and positivity for as long as you like. When you're ready, gently open your eyes and slowly return to your day.

Moon-time Journalling

When we are premenstrual, we are particularly intuitive and introspective. Journaling can be a powerful tool for tuning into your body and reflecting on your emotions, so that you can move into the month ahead with a clean slate. Here are some tips to help you get started if you've never tried this before.

Set aside dedicated time: Pick a time when you know you'll have a few minutes to yourself each day. This could be first thing in the morning or before bed. Try to make it a consistent time so that journaling becomes a habit and even write into your daily routine to make it a priority.

Choose a comfortable space: Find a quiet and comfortable spot where you can write without distractions. You might want to light a candle or diffuse some essential oils to help create a relaxing atmosphere. I'm a big fan of home altars, so maybe around your altar or home yoga space if you have one. If sitting in bed works for you, that's great too.

Use prompts: Sometimes it can be hard to know what to write about, so try using prompts or a journal to get started. Here are a few examples: How am I feeling physically? Emotionally? What goals do I have for the month ahead? What can I do to take care of myself this week?

Reflect on your menstrual cycle: Since you are premenstrual, this is a good time to reflect on your menstrual cycle and the past month. Note when you are expecting your period and any symptoms you may be experiencing. Pay attention to any patterns or changes you notice from month to month.

Practice self-compassion: It's important to be kind and gentle with yourself, especially when you are premenstrual. Use your journal to practice self-compassion by writing down affirmations and positive self-talk. Remind yourself of all the reasons why you are freaking awesome.

The goal of journaling is not to be perfect or to have a certain outcome, but to create a space for reflection and self-care. By taking the time to tune into your body and reflect on your emotions, you can set yourself up for a rejuvenating and fulfilling month ahead.

9. Where's My Libido? Yoga, Orgasms and Your Sex Life in Perimenopause

Why You Need Orgasms in Your Life

I know that sex may be the last thing on your mind. Fluctuating hormones, crazy mood swings and a 'withering' vagina. Extreme fatigue, discomfort and being stunned by the new modus-operandi of life, all contribute to pushing sex and orgasms to the bottom of our agendas. Not exactly 'hot stuff'. Yoga to the rescue once again, ladies!

However, I want to talk to you about the importance of orgasms (alone or with a partner) as they have huge benefits for all of us, especially during perimenopause! If you feel in need of some motivation as to why you should begin to explore that aspect of your life again, alone or with your special someone, read on.

Life without orgasms is just not great. Even if we are tired, bedraggled and feeling like shit, a 'little death' (as the French refers to orgasms) can bring us back to life with tons of health benefits. Not only do orgasms make for a happy lady, but a more patient, calm and balanced woman overall.

Orgasm is not only the crowning of a successful and highly pleasurable session of sex with your partner but something that could and absolutely should be achieved every day, even by yourself! With thousands of women across the world failing to ever reach orgasm (anorgasmia), it's important to look at why we even need the Big O in our lives at all.

Let's Look at What Orgasms Can Do for You

Orgasms Make You Feel Great Even When You're Not in The Middle of One

Orgasm is not limited in scope to making you feel good for five minutes before falling asleep. Science has shown that frequent sex and orgasms are very important to the general well-being and health of everyone. The more frequently you orgasm, the better you will feel on both a physical and psychological level.

Oxytocin is that magical hormone that rushes through the body when we first fall in love. Oxytocin can take us to the dizzy heights of a love sickness that makes food and sleep seem so much less important than looking into the eyes of our newfound love.

The hormone also plays an important part in sexual arousal and is released when you have an orgasm. It's important in nonsexual relationships too, and the presence of the hormone has been shown to increase trust, generosity and cooperation. The more oxytocin we release, the happier, relaxed and generally blissed out we become. Orgasms = Oxytocin. Do we need any more reasons?

Orgasms Release Stress and Tension

In a similar vein, perimenopause can cause nervous tension and stress. Just as jobs and relationships take their toll on mental balance, so do all these physical and emotional changes. Sex and orgasms are a chance for these tensions to be released. Thus, the mind uses orgasm to flush the tensions out of the system and replace them with the delicious relaxation that comes with the pleasure of the Big O.

It's Better Than Paracetamol for Killing Pain

Don't let your headaches get in the way. What our partners often don't realise is that headaches are often a woman's way of saying, 'You have to try harder', or 'I'd rather just sleep thank you'. The pleasure brought by orgasm is the result of a discharge of endorphins into the brain. No headache can survive the attack of pleasure flooding the brain and the calming effect it has. So, if the headache, fatigue or even insomnia is genuine, an orgasm can even help with this.

The Big O Before Bedtime Helps You Sleep

The best thing to do after disentangling from your lover's tender embrace is, of course, to slip into a deep sleep. The combined exertion of sex and relaxation brought by orgasm is the perfect replacement for any sleeping pill. Even if full sex is not back on the menu, take time to bring yourself to climax. This little extra will help you sleep soundly until it's time to get up with the baby. Instead of reaching out for a bottle of sleeping pills, you would be better off reaching out for the partner lying in the bed next to you or for your favourite sex toy (try a yoni egg for extra pelvic floor rejuvenation also). It's a perfectly natural solution that I heartily recommend.

Orgasms Curb Your Appetite (for food!)

Aside from releasing endorphins into the brain, sexual stimulation also activates the production of phenethylamine, an amphetamine secreted by the body which is thought to play a role in the regulation of appetite. Of course, sex is not meant to replace a healthy diet, but it seems to go some way toward helping you reign in those food cravings, and it does burn some calories. Cravings and overeating can go with the territory of perimenopause also, and orgasms will help to contain this. In fact, sex even burns more calories per minute than tennis. Fact.

Your Heart Needs Orgasms!

The number of scientific studies showing that frequent orgasms are good for one's health is testimony to the key role played by a successful sex life in the physical and mental health of all women. Heart health for women post-menopause can be a big issue, so let's get as many orgasms in now as possible. Aside from the fact that increased heart rate and heavy breathing keep the circulatory system in shape and make oxygen circulate through the body, sex has other benefits.

A study published in Psychosomatic Medicine in 1976 showed that failure to reach orgasm harms the cardiovascular health of women. Doctor Winnifred Cutler, a specialist in endocrinology, found that women who have sex at least once a week are more likely to have less painful menstrual cycles and higher levels of oestrogen in their blood. Healthy levels of oestrogen help keep the cardiovascular system in shape, fight cholesterol and keep the skin supple.

That's a great idea, if only I had time for orgasms.

Now, you have all the reasons you need to reintroduce orgasms into your life. Don't be put off by lack of time or privacy. Try using a yoni egg around the house during the day or in the evening after work. Not only will this rejuvenate the pelvic floor, but it will strengthen and tighten the vaginal canal and bring back sensitivity, which you may have lost or numbed through a lack of attention over the years. Don't feel bad about taking this time for yourself. This is the time to re-own your body and discover how it has changed and embrace this.

Life without orgasms is just not living up to its full potential. Even women that are having orgasms find them infrequent, short, sharp and well, basic. Let me explain how yoga can help improve your core strength, well-being and even your orgasm.

How Can Yoga Improve My Libido?

Let me explain. The body's core—which includes the abdominal, lower back, pelvis, and hip area (known as the *Hara* or life centre in women)—is considered in traditional medicine to be the most vital part of the body. The core is where the body's centre of gravity is located, and the muscles in this area work together to provide stability to the body. The core aims to bring force, power and stability from the legs to the upper body, and vice versa. At YogaBellies, we call this key area the BAPs (the back, abs and pelvic floor), and the integrity of the BAPs is essential for every woman's health throughout life.

Many of the body's core muscles cannot be seen because they are hidden underneath other muscles. It's widely known that a strong core makes it easier to practise yoga arm balances and inversions and other strength-based activities. The core has many other important roles, including improving your overall well-being and sexual health. Yoga Asana, focus on strengthening this core or 'Hara'.

Get to The Core of It

Now, our core suffers during perimenopause too, we know this. Practising a core-focused yoga practice, at least once a week, helps to protect the spinal cord and enriches and stimulates many of our organs. Yoga will help you develop a healthy body, increase your lifespan, become relaxed and even have a better sex life!

Studies show that practising yoga helps promote increased energy levels, improved confidence and self-esteem and increased testosterone levels. Practising Yoga Asana acts almost as a 'massage' for the internal organs, enabling the body's internal systems to function properly. Both Eastern and Western medicine agree on the benefits of a well-developed and strengthened core.

According to Eastern Medicine, the core is the centre of all human energy. These principles believe that the core is the source of the 'chi'—the power within. The 'chi' is responsible for self-healing, self-recovery and self-realisation. Chinese beliefs add that this power is a life force and is present in every living thing. The 'chi' flows in the body through channels called meridians and gives the body life nourishment and energy. The chi can be developed by meditation, visualisation and breathing. Core strength is so important for women. Incorporating core-focused asana in your yoga practice will increase strength, avoid muscle injury and improve your posture and balance.

Orgasms During Yoga?

The 2014 National Survey of Sexual Health and Behaviour (NSSHB) in the USA looked at 2,000 Americans and their sex lives. They found that around 10% of men and women reported experiencing an orgasm from exercise, and even more reported getting turned on while working out. For women, 'coregasms' were most likely to happen during core-specific exercises such as yoga. As if we needed more of a reason to go to do yoga.

Yoga to Improve Your Sex Life Every Day

Although the exact reason for core asana enhancing and even bringing on orgasms is still unclear, it is believed that it's possible that those core muscles are working together with the nerve pathways and the pelvic floor to create orgasmic sensations during or after your yoga practice. Another theory is that it could be that your tired, wobbly core muscles create some type of inner stimulation that engages other nearby organs and creates these incredibly intense sensations.

No need to worry about rocking the Big O in a yoga class though: these enlightening studies identified that more people report exercise-induced arousal and improved orgasms after their yoga practice than actual core exercise-induced orgasms.

My Top Yoga Tips for Improving Your Sex Life Mid-Life

So, this is all very well, but what specifically should we focus on during our yoga practice to improve our Big O or general libido, afterwards?

You could begin with a flowing dynamic yoga practice which doubles as your cardio. Try multiple repetitions of dynamic sun salutations (Surya Namaskar A and B) to build heat in the body and increase the heart rate. Aim to engage the sympathetic nervous system before starting core-specific exercises.

Focus on core-specific asana such as *Chaturanga Dandasana* (4-legged stag pose/plank); *Navasana* (boat pose); *Uttkatasana* (Chair pose) and Bakkasana (Crow pose).

Multiple repetitions will really fatigue your core, essential for coregasms.

Bring *Vinyasa* (flow) or sun salutations back into the middle of your practice to mix it up. The studies showed that mixing up cardio with weight-bearing and core-strengthening exercises, helped to improve orgasm potential.

Bring your attention to the breath and relax. Allow yourself to enjoy your yoga practice as a moving meditation, meeting each movement with an inhale or exhale. *Ujjayi* breathing is perfect for this purpose.

Go forth and enjoy a beautiful, blissful yoga practice and intensified orgasms lovelies!

Yoga and Meditation to Heighten Your Libido

This is a cracking and very simple yoga sequence for getting those fires burning again, which can be particularly useful if you've been suffering from anxiety, low mood or discomfort because of vaginal dryness. It's going to help increase your libido and interest in all things sexual during this time. Check out the Yoni Yoga sequences if this is an area of special concern for you.

Sukkhasana (Easy pose): Sit cross-legged with a straight spine, hands on the knees or in chin mudra. Easy pose sets the scene for a calm mind and improves blood flow to the pelvic region.

Baddha Konasana (Butterfly pose): Bring the soles of the feet together and gently flap the knees up and down. This pose stimulates the reproductive organs and helps relieve stress and releases emotional pain held in the hips.

Sethu Bandasana (Bridge pose): Lie on your back with knees bent, feet hip-distance apart, and lift your hips towards the ceiling. Bridge increases blood flow to the pelvic area, strengthens the pelvic floor muscles, and helps alleviate stress and fatigue.

Usttrasana (Camel pose): Kneel with your legs hip-distance apart, place your hands on your lower back, and arch your back as you reach your hands back towards your heels. This pose improves blood flow to the pelvic area, helps alleviate stress, and opens up the heart chakra.

Ardha Matsyendrasana (Half Lord of the Fishes pose): Sit with your legs extended, cross your left foot over your right thigh, and place your right hand on your left knee as you twist to the left. Repeat on the other side. This pose helps stimulate the reproductive organs, improves digestion, and increases blood flow to the pelvic area.

Viparitta Kirani (Legs up the wall pose): Lie on your back with your legs extended up the wall. Legs up the wall helps improve blood flow to the pelvic region, calms the mind, and alleviates stress and fatigue.

Savasana (Corpse pose): Lie on your back with your arms and legs extended, palms facing up. Close your eyes and relax your body completely. Savasana is the ultimate relaxation posture.

Wild Woman Meditation to Keep Those Fires Burning:

This meditation will help you increase your libido and to reconnect with your sexuality by embodying the archetype of the 'Wild Woman:'

Begin by finding a comfortable seated position. You can sit on the floor with your legs crossed, or in a chair with your feet flat on the ground. Rest your hands on your knees or in your lap.

Take a few deep breaths, inhaling through your nose and exhaling through your mouth. With each exhale, release any tension or stress you may be holding in your body.

Close your eyes and bring your attention to your breath. Notice the sensation of the breath moving in and out of your body.

As you continue to breathe deeply, visualise yourself stepping into the archetype of the Enchantress. The Enchantress is a sensual and alluring figure, who is in touch with her body and her desires. Imagine that you are embodying this archetype - feel her power and her sensuality. The Wild Woman is a free spirit, who is in touch with her primal instincts and her sexuality. Imagine that you are embodying this archetype - feel her wildness and her passion.

> *I am worthy of pleasure and joy in my life.*
>
> *My body is strong, healthy, and vibrant.*

I embrace my sexuality and sensuality with confidence and self-love.

I am open to new experiences and new ways of experiencing pleasure and intimacy.

I am grateful for the opportunity to connect with my body and my sexuality in a positive way.

As you hold the Enchantress in your mind, allow yourself to connect with your own sensuality and sexuality. Allow yourself to feel desire and pleasure in your body.

Take a few more deep breaths, then when you're ready, slowly open your eyes.

Take a moment to notice how you feel. You may feel more connected to your body and your desires, and more open to experiencing pleasure and intimacy.

This meditation can be practised regularly to help you connect with your own sensuality and increase your libido during perimenopause. Remember, it is important to listen to your body and only engage in sexual activity that feels comfortable and enjoyable for you.

10. Incorporating Yoga into Your Daily Routine

Creating a daily routine that includes the key elements of the YogaPause sadhana, can be a really powerful tool for managing the demands of perimenopause life. The key to success is consistency, and you should commit to setting aside dedicated time each day to do a variation of each of these things. Change it up throughout the month and honour your body when it tells you that this practice is no longer working or that you need to try something new.

Here is some guidance on how to create a daily schedule that includes a physical yoga practice, breathing techniques, mindfulness and meditation, relaxation and community.

Step 1: Assess Your Needs

The first step is to assess your needs. What symptoms are you experiencing? What areas of your life are most affected by perimenopause and ageing? What do you hope to achieve through yoga, breathing techniques, meditation and movement? Yoga is not about goals, it's about the journey, but it's good to have something to focus on. For example, are you here mostly because of low mood and anxiety or is it something physical? Or both! By answering these questions honestly, you'll have a clearer understanding of what you need and what you're hoping to achieve from changing your lifestyle.

Step 2: Establish a Realistic Routine

Once you know what you need, the next step is to get together your routine. Start with a time frame that works best for you. Some of us prefer to practise first thing in the morning; others prefer to practise in the evening before bed. Choose a time when you're least likely to be disturbed, and make sure you allow yourself enough time for each practice. If you want a ready-made plan, pop over to the YogaBellies website and check out my 'Naturally' Fabulous Over 40 programme, which does all of the hard work for you.

Step 3: Choose Your Practices

The next step is to choose the yoga, breathing techniques, meditation and movement practices that best meet your needs. There are many different practices to choose from, so it's important to select the ones that resonate with you and suit your needs, on any given day. Remember this can change based on what kind of day/week you're having, what's going on in your life and where you are in your menstrual cycle (if you're still able to track it!). Some common practices you should consider are obviously physical yoga postures, pranayama (yoga breathing techniques), mindfulness meditation and other kinds of gentle movement too, like dancing, walking, or jogging. Refer to the sadhana for ideas and inspiration of what to include.

Step 4: Practise Consistently

Consistency is key to getting into the swing of a daily routine. Now remember, consistency for a woman looks different than it does for a man. We are not linear beings, we're cyclical. We look and feel different every day of the month because of our fluctuating hormones and energetic highs and lows. Consistency as a woman means being aware of where you are in your cycle and honouring that. You can still make a 'routine' within that and allow yourself to be as flexible as necessary. If you miss a day, don't worry, simply get back on track the next day or give your body what it needs on that particular day.

Step 5: Adjust as Needed

As your needs change over time, be open to adjusting your yoga practice and routine. Things will change for all the reasons mentioned previously. For example, you may find that you need to practise for a shorter or longer period, or that you need to switch to a different type of practice or practise for longer or even start adding in weights for more of a challenge.

All this is ok! Be open to making changes and listening to what your body and soul need on any given day.

My example weekly wellness schedule

This is an example schedule of what a typical week could look like for you. It incorporates all the key wellness practices we've discussed, but again, remember that it's YOUR schedule so mix it up as you want to and fit it into a format that works for you. I like to get everything in during the day because I'm a morning body and go to bed at 8 or 9 pm most nights, but if you're a night owl, switch it around. If it doesn't feel good, the chances are you won't stick to it.

Monday:

- Morning: Gentle YogaPause practice for 30 minutes, focusing on stretching and opening up the body. Incorporate poses such as Downward-Facing Dog, Cat-Cow and Child's Pose to help release tension and stress.

- Mid-morning: 10-minute breathing technique to help calm the mind and reduce stress levels. Try Nadi Shodhana—or Alternate Nostril Breathing—where you breathe in and out through one nostril at a time.

- Afternoon: 30-minute meditation practice, focusing on mindfulness and relaxation. Try a guided meditation, such as a body scan or a visualisation exercise, to help you connect with your breath and calm your mind.

- Late afternoon: 30-minute walk in nature, if possible, to help boost mood and increase physical activity.

Tuesday:

- Morning: Dynamic YogaPause practice for 45 minutes, focusing on strengthening and toning the body. Incorporate poses such as Warrior II, Triangle and Warrior III, to help build muscle and improve balance.

- Mid-morning: 10-minute breathing technique to help energise the body and improve circulation. Try Kapalabhati, or Skull Shining Breath, where you rapidly contract and release the abdominal muscles.

- Afternoon: 30-minute meditation practice, focusing on gratitude and positive affirmations. Try repeating affirmations such as 'I am worthy; I am loved, and I am enough' to help build self-esteem and boost mood.

- Late afternoon: 30-minute walk or light jog to help improve cardiovascular health and release endorphins.

Wednesday:

- Morning: Restorative yoga practice for 30 minutes, focusing on relaxation and release. Incorporate poses such as Supported Bridge, Reclining Bound Angle and Legs Up the Wall, to help reduce stress and tension.

- Mid-morning: 10-minute breathing technique to help release tension and improve sleep quality. Try Ujjayi, or Victorious Breath, where you slow down the breath and make a soft, ocean-like sound in the back of your throat.

- Afternoon: 30-minute meditation practice, focusing on self-compassion and self-love. Try repeating affirmations such as 'I am kind to myself; I am gentle with myself, and I am deserving of love and care' to help build self-esteem and boost mood.

- Late afternoon: 30-minute Yoga Nidra practice, focusing on deep relaxation and release.

Thursday:

- Morning: YogaPause practice for 45 minutes, focusing on balance and stability. Incorporate poses such as Tree Pose, Eagle Pose and Half-Moon, to help build strength and improve balance.

- Mid-morning: 10-minute breathing technique to help reduce stress and anxiety. Try Brahmarri, or Bee Breath, where you hum like a bee to help calm the mind and reduce tension.

- Afternoon: 30-minute meditation practice, focusing on compassion and kindness. Try repeating affirmations such as 'I am kind to others. I am gentle with others', to help build self-esteem and boost mood.

- Late afternoon: 30-minute Yoga Nidra practice, focusing on deep relaxation and release. Try repeating affirmations such as 'I am kind; I am compassionate, and I spread love and kindness wherever I go' to help build a positive mindset and improve relationships.

- Late afternoon: 30-minute walk or light hike to enjoy nature and get some fresh air.

Friday:

- Morning: Gentle vinyasa yoga practice for 60 minutes, focusing on fluid movements and increased heart rate. Incorporate poses such as Sun Salutations, Warrior I and Chair Pose, to help increase cardiovascular health and improve strength.

- Mid-morning: 10-minute breathing technique to help improve focus and concentration. Try Trattaka, or Candle Gazing, where you gaze at a small flame to help calm the mind and improve focus.

- Afternoon: 30-minute meditation practice, focusing on visualisation and manifestation. Try visualising your goals and desires, and repeating affirmations such as 'I am capable; I am worthy, and I am on the path to success' to help build confidence and motivation.

- Late afternoon: 30-minute walk or dance session to improve mood and release endorphins.

Saturday:

- Morning: YogaPause Strong practice for 75 minutes, focusing on strength and endurance. Incorporate poses such as Plank Pose, Chaturanga and Upward-Facing Dog, to help build upper body strength and improve core stability.

- Mid-morning: 10-minute breathing technique to help reduce anxiety and improve mood. Try Pranayama, or Control of Life Force Breath, where you practise slow, deep breathing to help regulate the nervous system.

- Afternoon: 30-minute meditation practice, focusing on self-reflection and personal growth. Try journaling or reflection exercises to help identify areas of growth and areas for improvement.

- Late afternoon: 30-minute walk or light jog to improve cardiovascular health and release endorphins.

Remember, this is just an example schedule and can be modified to suit your individual preferences. The most important thing is to make time for self-care and to incorporate practices that help you manage the physical and emotional changes of perimenopause. So, find what works best for you and make it a regular part of your daily life.

11. Happy Mind: Happy Life

The connection between mindset and health is well established, with countless studies showing that a positive outlook can have a huge impact on our mental well-being and on our physical health. This is especially true when our body is undergoing drastic changes and our hormones are working against our ability to process these changes rationally.

Developing a positive mindset towards ageing also means focusing on the things that bring you real happiness and fulfilment. This could be spending time with your friends and loved ones, pursuing that hobby you didn't have time to take up when the kids were babies or enjoying physical activity that genuinely makes you feel good. By prioritising these things and making time for YOU every day, you'll find a renewed enthusiasm for life and the little things.

Ageing and the Patriarchy

Before we delve into how patriarchy and religious doctrines eroded the authority of older women, it's important to understand the Crone archetype. The term 'Crone' represents a woman who has moved past middle age and who embodies wisdom, knowledge, and represents a life fully lived. Contrary to modern derogatory connotations associated with old age, the Crone was once considered a societal pillar, imparting wisdom and often serving as healers, advisors, and leaders.

The shift from a balanced or even matriarchal society to a patriarchal one didn't happen overnight either. In early human history, both men and women had roles that were essential for survival. Over time, as societies started to build around agriculture rather than hunting and gathering, property and lineage began to hold more importance. Men, being physically stronger, became protectors of property, leading to increased power and eventually forming patriarchal societies.

In the patriarchy's quest for dominance, religion became a tool to institutionalize male authority. Biblical stories like 'Adam and Eve' instigated the perception that women were not only secondary but also the originators of sin. Older women, with their wisdom and knowledge, became particular targets. Why? Because their wisdom was a threat to the established order.

In many religious texts, older women were either completely invisible or portrayed as witches, hags, or temptresses. They were no longer the wise Crones but caricatures to be avoided or vilified. The 'Witch Trials' that happened in medieval Europe can be viewed as an extreme form of institutionalized ageism and misogyny, where older women, often the wise women of the community, were accused of witchcraft and brutally executed.

One of the most obvious ways the patriarchy dissolved the power of the Crone was by replacing goddess worship with male gods. For example, the triple goddess concept, which included the Maiden, Mother, (Enchantress) and Crone, was gradually overshadowed by the worship of singular male gods who were omnipotent. The Crone goddesses who were previously revered for their wisdom and life-giving and taking capabilities were downgraded to lesser deities or forgotten altogether.

For centuries, patriarchal culture has defined women's worth based on youth, beauty and fertility. Women were expected to conform to rigid standards of being 'attractive' to be child-bearers and to stay at home as wives and mothers. These roles were previously seen as our only path to fulfilment and happiness while any deviation from this was considered deviant or even sinful in some cultures.

Today, older women often find themselves at the margins of society: invisible in the media, passed over for jobs, and disregarded in social situations. The power of age and wisdom, particularly in women, is rarely celebrated. What's more, women's health issues surrounding menopause and ageing are under-researched and stigmatized, which can be traced back to this patriarchal devaluation of the older woman.

The patriarchy's obsession with youth and beauty has continued to result in unrealistic and unattainable standards that have caused all of us to suffer from body image issues, low self-esteem, and anxiety. Add to this, fashion magazines and social media, we've been bombarded with images of pin-thin models and celebrities with perfectly toned bodies, flawless skin and unrealistic proportions. This insane, toxic beauty culture has led many of us to unhealthy habits, like extreme and/or yo-yo dieting, plastic surgery and even eating disorders. N.B., I have no issue with surgery so long as the woman in question is not doing it for anyone other than herself. As we continue to speak out on this BS and demand change, this beauty ideal is slowly starting to lose its grip.

The fertile 'maiden' archetype has long been seen as the pinnacle of feminine beauty and the 'mother' as fulfilling her role as a woman and life-giver. So, what happens when we don't or no longer fall into these categories? What's next?

The patriarchy's emphasis on fertility has always been a source of massive pressure and anxiety for women. The expectation that we should all be able to bear children has led many of us to feelings of inadequacy and shame if we're unable or choose not to have children. I have one son and have lost multiple pregnancies and I've heard so many times, "You can't just have one!" Even as women ourselves, sensitivity around other women's parenting choices and fertility challenges is still low. Moreover, the assumption that as women we are solely responsible for child-rearing and domestic duties has limited our professional opportunities and hindered our economic independence. However, as more women move into the workforce and become financially independent, this expectation is to some extent, beginning to shift.

As we move (slowly) towards a more equal and inclusive society, women are increasingly valued for our intelligence, creativity and leadership skills. Our voices and perspectives are finally being heard in all areas of life, from politics to business, and from the arts to technology. This recognition of our unique and diverse talents and capabilities is breaking down those traditional barriers that have kept us in narrow, stereotypical roles.

There are so many women who are celebrated for their accomplishments and contributions, regardless of their age or appearance. Women like Ruth Bader Ginsburg, Angela Merkel and Malala Yousafzai have become powerful symbols of female leadership and inspiration for women all over the world. These incredible women embody the idea that women's worth is not limited by their youth, beauty or fertility, but rather by their intelligence, compassion and strength, exactly as it should be.

So let's not end this chapter on a bleak note. The Crone is making a comeback, albeit slowly, thanks to the rise of modern spirituality and efforts to redefine age and femininity. Women are reclaiming this life stage as one of empowerment, wisdom, and, dare we say, rebellion.

Everyday Mindfulness and Impermanence

Mindfulness is the practice of being present and fully engaged in the current moment. It involves paying attention to your thoughts, emotions and physical sensations without judgement. Meditation, on the other hand, is a specific technique used to train the mind to focus and relax.

Practising mindfulness can help us better understand and accept the impermanent nature of reality. Change is a natural part of life that can bring both positive and negative emotions and mindfulness can help us approach these with more grace and ease. In Buddhism, impermanence means that all things, including our thoughts and experiences, are transient and subject to change: the good times come, and the bad times go. When I first converted to Buddhism, the concept of the Wheel of Life really resonated with me. Also known as the Bhavacakra, it's a symbolic representation of samsara, the cycle of birth, death, and rebirth. The wheel is divided into six realms, each representing a different state of existence, from the heavenly realm to the hell realm. Regardless of your religious preferences, stick with me, as this is a valuable concept.

An important aspect of the Wheel of Life is the concept of impermanence, which is central to Buddhist philosophy. The wheel is constantly turning, representing the impermanent and ever-changing nature of our earthly existence. According to Buddhist teachings, everything in the world is impermanent, from our thoughts and emotions to the physical objects around us. Nothing lasts forever, and clinging to things that are impermanent (like money and cellulite-free bodies) can only lead to suffering.

For me, it's a reminder that all things are impermanent and that this cycle is an opportunity to learn and grow. By understanding the impermanent nature of our existence, we can cultivate a sense of detachment and learn to let go of attachments that cause suffering. That could be attachment to youth or fertility or wrinkle-free skin. By understanding that this is all part of the journey, we can let it go.

The wheel reminds us that everything is constantly changing, and that impermanence is a natural and inevitable part of life. By embracing impermanence and learning to let go, we can cultivate a sense of contentment and freedom from this constant suffering or 'grasping' at things we can never keep hold of.

It really helped me reevaluate my priorities in life and consider what was important and what was actually worth worrying about. Do I really want to spend the next 40 years being sad about the fact that I no longer look the way I did when I was 20? Absolutely not.

By actively practising mindfulness, we become more aware and accepting of this impermanence. Studies (because we love a bit of evidence) have shown that a consistent mindfulness practice can improve our ability to cope with difficult experiences, including reminders of our own mortality. For those of us in midlife, the concept of impermanence is so relevant and helpful if we can truly grasp its meaning.

When people hear about mindfulness, they often think of long periods sitting cross-legged in silent meditation. But did you know that there are other ways to practise mindfulness just going about your everyday business? Research has shown that even short, informal mindfulness practices can have huge benefits for us as women.

Formal mindfulness practices refer to things like setting aside time for meditation, like doing body scans, sitting meditations or mindful movement such as yoga. Informal mindfulness practice is all about infusing mindfulness into your daily routine, like being mindful when you're washing the dishes, taking a walk through the park, talking to people at work or even something as basic as showering or eating your lunch. By approaching run-of-the-mill activities with intentionality and awareness, you can enhance your state of ongoing mindfulness.

Studies have also found that informal mindfulness practices are more important for your well-being and psychological flexibility than the formal practices. So, don't worry if you don't have a lot of time for sitting meditation. Just taking a few mindful moments throughout your day can make a significant difference to being fully present in your life.

Even brief mindfulness practices can immediately affect your mood, stress levels and anxiety. For example, a 20-minute meditation session can significantly lower stress responses. And even just 5–10 minutes of daily practice can help you to feel less anxious.

So, whether you have a lot of time or just a few minutes, there are tons of simple ways that you can incorporate mindfulness into your life. We'll explore some basic mindfulness and meditation practices that may be helpful during perimenopause.

Mindful breathing: Mindful breathing is a super simple practice that simply involves paying attention to your breath. Sit comfortably, close your eyes and take a few deep breaths. Then, focus your attention on your breath as it moves in and out of your body. Notice the sensation of the breath as it enters and leaves your nostrils, and how your chest and abdomen rise and fall. If your mind wanders, gently bring your attention back to your breath.

Body scan meditation: Body scan meditation involves systematically scanning through each part of your body, bringing awareness to any sensations you feel. Lie down or sit comfortably, close your eyes and start by focusing on your breath. Then, bring your attention to your toes and slowly work your way up through your body, noticing any sensations you feel. This practice can be especially helpful in reducing physical tension and promoting relaxation.

Loving-kindness meditation: Loving-kindness meditation involves generating feelings of love, compassion and well-wishes towards yourself and others. Sit comfortably, close your eyes, and take a few deep breaths. Then, bring to mind someone you care about and silently repeat the following phrases to yourself:

May you be happy

May you be healthy

May you be safe

May you be at peace

Repeat these phrases, either for the same person or different people, focusing on generating feelings of kindness and compassion.

Mindful Walking or Walking Meditation: Mindful walking involves paying attention to your body and the environment around you as you walk. Find a quiet place to walk and start by bringing your attention to your feet. Notice the sensation of your feet making contact with the ground, the movement of your legs and your arms swinging by your side. Then, bring your attention to your surroundings, noticing the colours, shapes and sounds around you.

Affirmations

I freaking love affirmations. So simple and effective. Positive affirmations are short, powerful statements that can help us reprogramme our thoughts and beliefs. By repeating these affirmations regularly, we can train our brains to focus on the good in our lives and let go of the bs. Here are some examples of positive affirmations that can help you navigate perimenopause:

I trust my body to know what it needs.

I am strong, resilient and capable of handling any challenge.

I release all fears and worries about the future.

I am grateful for the wisdom that comes with age.

I honour my body's natural rhythms and cycles.

I am at peace with the changes happening within me.

I choose to focus on the positive aspects of my life.

I am deserving of love, respect and happiness.

I am surrounded by people who support and uplift me.

I am open to new experiences and opportunities.

You can use these affirmations in different ways. You can write them down on post-it notes and stick them on your mirror, fridge or computer screen. You can also repeat them to yourself as you go about your day, especially when you feel stressed or overwhelmed. Another option is to create a vision board or a journal where you can write down your favourite affirmations and add images that inspire you.

Remember, positive affirmations are not a magic solution to all of your problems, but they can help you shift your focus and find more meaning in your life. So, take a deep breath, repeat your favourite affirmation and let the magic unfold!

Sankalpa

Sankalpa is a Sanskrit term that means 'a resolution or intention formed in the heart or mind'. It's a powerful tool used in the practice of Yoga Nidra—a form of guided meditation that promotes deep relaxation and inner awareness. I have tons of these on my YouTube channel and on the podcast too if you'd like to listen to an audio version. In Yoga Nidra, the Sankalpa is a positive statement that aligns with our deepest desires and helps us connect with our true nature. It's a statement that we repeat to ourselves at the beginning and end of the practice, to plant it in our subconscious mind.

During perimenopause, we can feel really disconnected from our changing bodies and uncertain about the future. We may feel like we're losing our sense of identity. This is where the practice of Sankalpa can be super powerful. By setting a positive intention and repeating it regularly, we can shift our focus from what we don't want to what we do want. We can connect with our inner wisdom and find the strength and resilience to face the challenges of perimenopause.

Here's how to create a Sankalpa:

- Find a quiet and comfortable place where you can sit or lie down without interruption.

- Take a few deep breaths and allow yourself to relax.

- Close your eyes and visualise yourself in a peaceful and serene place, such as a beach or a forest.

- Ask yourself, 'What is my deepest desire for this stage of my life?'

- Listen to your heart and allow a positive statement to arise. It could be something like, 'I am strong and capable of handling anything that comes my way,' or 'I embrace the changes in my body and trust the natural process of life.'

- Repeat this statement to yourself three times, slowly and with conviction.

- Visualise your Sankalpa taking root in your heart and spreading throughout your body.

- When you're ready to end your practice, take a few more deep breaths and open your eyes.

Remember, your Sankalpa is a personal statement that reflects your unique needs and aspirations. You can adjust it as you need, depending on where you are in your menopause journey. The key is to choose a statement that resonates with you and feels true to your heart. With regular practice, your Sankalpa can become a guiding light that helps you stay centred and focused, no matter what challenges come your way.

These are just a few examples of mindfulness and meditation practices that can be helpful during perimenopause, but there are so many out there to explore.

12. Yoga and Positivity

The fact is that yoga literally makes you radiate positivity. The 'love hormone' Oxytocin helps you to relax and reduces blood pressure and cortisol levels, and Yoga is well recognised as one of the best ways to release this amazing hormone and built-in anti-stress mechanism.

When the various limbs of yoga are practised, oxytocin is released. Deep breathing warms the body, and warmth is one of the key elements that allow us to release oxytocin. By taking the body through the practice of yoga asana (postures), we warm the muscles and joints and make the physical body more comfortable and relaxed. By then continuing the practice with savasana (deep relaxation) and meditation, we encourage the production of oxytocin even further.

What is Oxytocin?

Oxytocin is that magical hormone that rushes through the body when we first fall in love. Oxytocin can take us to the dizzy heights of a love sickness that makes food and sleep seem so much less important than looking into the eyes of our newfound love.

Some of oxytocin's main functions are to prepare the female body for childbirth, stimulate milk production and 'let down' so that the baby can nurse and encourage the bond between mum and her new-born baby.

The hormone also plays an important part in sexual arousal and is released when you have an orgasm. It's important in nonsexual relationships too and the presence of the hormone has been shown to increase trust, generosity and cooperation.

Why Does Yoga Make You Happy?

Yogic breathing (of course!). When the vagus nerve is inflamed, your breathing becomes shallower. Your body has gone into fight or flight mode, and you have started to panic. Stop right here and allow yourself to breathe deeply. Pranayama (or yogic breathing) encourages us to take time to just stop and focus on the breath.

This time of life has so many huge physical, emotional, and environmental changes that can be difficult to adapt to. Taking some time each week to just breathe during yoga class, bringing your attention to the breath, focusing on the breath alone and not worrying about anything else, can allow oxytocin to be released and deepen that relaxation. Slow steady breathing is all that you need. Sometimes, we get so caught up in 'getting the posture' that we forget to breathe. Check yourself and make sure you ARE actually breathing (you'd be surprised).

Warming the body through the practice of Asana

It is important to warm the body before undertaking the physical practice of yoga (asana) so as not to damage any joints and to ease the body gently into the postures. This is especially important for pregnant and post-natal women, whose bodies are and have undergone physical stress and growth over time. During the practice of asana and pranayama, the body generates heat and warms the body inside and out. Bonus?

When we are warm and relaxed, the body releases more oxytocin.

Chilling in Savasana

At the end of class or your practice, don't just jump up and run out of class. Savasana, deep relaxation, at the end of class is your reward for all your hard effort earlier on. Learn to enjoy the relaxation, be aware of any random thoughts that go through your mind—and just let them go. This is known as 'monkey mind'. What will I have for dinner? What did she mean by that? Acknowledge these meaningless thoughts and really take time for yourself. Just focus on the life force—the breath. That's all you need to do. And enjoy the scrummy feeling of the copious oxytocin rushing through your body. Sigh.

Why is Oxytocin so important for women

In a study of sixty-five women with depression and anxiety, the 34 women who took a yoga class twice a week for two months showed a significant decrease in depression and anxiety symptoms, compared to the 31 women who were not in the class.

Pain Relief

Oxytocin helps us when we're in pain as well as providing pain-relieving endorphins. A notable example of this is giving birth. If you had a drug-free birth, you'll be familiar with the body's natural painkillers. As soon as the baby is born, it makes mum fall in love in the greatest way possible, with their new-born baby.

In the first few moments after giving birth, a mother receives the largest rush of oxytocin that she will ever experience in her lifetime.

Mood swings and Depression

Yoga helps to balance hormones and stabilises the endocrine system. By practising yogic relaxation, we can balance cortical activities and the nervous and endocrine systems, reducing the body's reaction to stress. As a result, the body produces less adrenaline, noradrenaline and cortisol—all stress hormones—and mum feels much more balanced and stressed-free.

Also, depression studies indicate clinical depression alleviates by half if only we can talk to a friend who listens to us, and oxytocin is shown to increase when we receive empathy. The social aspects of getting out to yoga classes are important for socialising with other women going through the same life experiences.

Gratitude

Another important aspect of developing a positive perimenopause mindset (PPM!) is practising gratitude. Taking time each day to reflect on the things you are grateful for can help shift your focus away from negative thoughts and toward a more positive outlook. For example, YES, your boobs may not be as perky as they used to be, but how much more confident and comfortable in your own body are you than when you were 20?

It turns out that science has also shown us that practising gratitude can have some pretty awesome benefits for our physical and mental health. When we practise gratitude, we're actively appreciating the things that sustain our lives, which can lead to a deeper sense of contentment. Research has found that people who practise gratitude tend to be happier, have more positive emotions and have better relationships with others. Plus, they're often more helpful and empathetic too!

One study conducted by Dr Philip Watkins in 2003 found that gratitude is linked to improved mood and overall well-being. And the cool thing is, these benefits aren't just limited to certain groups of people. Studies have also shown that more grateful people tend to have better physical health, engage in healthier activities and sleep better too! So, why not try incorporating a little gratitude into your life and see how it makes you feel? Try keeping a gratitude or cycle journal or taking a few minutes each day to meditate on the simple things that make you happy.

Write It Down

Journaling is basically a type of writing where you can reflect on your emotions, thoughts and behaviours. It's a terrific way to gain perspective on different situations. According to Dr James Pennebaker (1998), journaling can actually boost your immune system, improve your mood and even help you manage stress. Plus, it's been shown to help with symptoms of depression, and trauma and improve memory. How incredible is that? And it's not just for mental health. Journaling has also been linked to physical benefits like lowering blood pressure and strengthening the immune system.

As a woman going through midlife, journaling might be particularly helpful in managing other symptoms related to eating disorders, grief and anxiety. Plus, incorporating gratitude journaling can have some pretty amazing effects on your well-being, like reducing physical pain, improving sleep quality and increasing optimism. And by focusing on gratitude, you're also more likely to engage in kind and supportive behaviours towards others, which can expand your social support network.

Impermanence and Acceptance

Impermanence is a key teaching in mindfulness that emphasizes the constantly changing nature of everything around us. Something I'm sure you are very aware of right now! And it's particularly relevant to women going through midlife transitions, which can be quite a traumatic time if we don't have the right mindset.

Impermanence isn't all bad! In fact, it can be a valuable reminder of the many gifts that change can bring. As we embark on this new phase of life, we can approach it with more awareness, wisdom and grace. I wanted to share this with you because I honestly believe it's important to embrace change and all the possibilities it brings.

Right alongside impermanence is acceptance. Acceptance plays a vital role in our happiness. Accepting ourselves and whatever is happening around us doesn't mean we are passive or disconnected from reality. It's quite the opposite actually! It allows our minds to embrace reality for what it is with a deeper understanding. Mindful acceptance can help us regulate our emotions, reduce any pain, and negative feelings. Research has shown that having a non-judgmental attitude towards our experiences can even diminish the negative effects of low self-esteem on depression. Equanimity is another fantastic aspect of mindfulness, which encourages us to have an even-minded disposition towards everything we experience, no matter their origin or emotional nature.

Feeling the Love

It's important to surround yourself with positive people that make you feel good, whether that means spending time with supportive friends and family members or seeking out resources and female communities that align with your values, interests and life stage. This will help you stay motivated and inspired, even during times when you may be feeling shitty or overwhelmed.

Developing a positive mindset is not always easy, and it can take time and practice to make changes. However, the benefits of actively trying to not be a negative nelly are well worth the effort and can help you navigate the ups and downs of perimenopause a lot easier.

There are also specific yogic mindset strategies and philosophies that can be particularly helpful during perimenopause. For example, developing a sense of acceptance is a big deal. Mindfulness can help you stay present at the moment and focus on what you can control, rather than dwelling on the things you can't change (those boobs again unless you want to go under the knife!). This can be especially helpful when dealing with symptoms like hot flashes or mood swings, which can be difficult to manage.

It's important to remember that this time of life can also be an opportunity for growth, self-discovery and positive change. We'll explore ways to maintain a positive mindset for optimal wellness during perimenopause.

Why Getting Older Is Cool AF

As women, we constantly hear negative messages about ageing, particularly when it comes to life after forty. We've already discussed the fact that society tells us that we are no longer youthful, no longer beautiful and no longer desirable. However, I call bullshit on all of this. As you age, you begin to discover the incredible gifts that come with experience. Here are just a few amazing things about getting older that you may want to consider:

Increased Confidence: As we age, we become more comfortable in our own skin. We know who we are and what we want, and we are less likely to be swayed by other people's opinions or expectations.

We develop a 'don't give AF' attitude that we rarely held in our twenties. We're no longer trying to impress people, because we just don't care! This newfound confidence is our most powerful tool that allows us to take risks, try new things and stand up for ourselves.

Wisdom: With age comes wisdom, and this is especially true for women. We have lived through a lot of experiences, both good and bad, and we have learned valuable lessons along the way. We may have given birth, raised children, had multiple relationships or careers. We can draw on all of this to make better decisions and navigate life's challenges. By this point, we've encountered most of life's idiots and players and we're much more attuned to those people who are good or bad for our lives.

Stronger Relationships: As we age, we tend to focus more on the quality of our relationships rather than the quantity. In your twenties you may have had a huge gang of 'party pals,' but now your friendship circle is probably considerably smaller. We have learned to prioritise the people who matter most to us, and we are more willing to invest time and energy in building and maintaining strong, meaningful connections.

Greater Financial Stability: By the time we reach our 40s, many of us have established successful careers and built up a solid financial foundation. This financial stability gives us the freedom to pursue our passions, travel and enjoy the fruits of our labour. I also know that this can also be the time when many of us are getting divorced and if we've stayed home with the children, may not have the same career level as others or finances available. It's never too late to begin your dream career, now is the time to consider what you love, what you're good at and how you can make this your life's work. As I said before, do you really want to be doing something you hate for the next 20 years?

Better Health: While ageing can come with its own challenges, many of us find that we become more health conscious as we get older. We tend to pay more attention to what we eat, how much we exercise, how much sleep we get and how we manage stress, which can lead to better overall health and longevity. Also, when weight maintenance and high energy levels are no longer a given, we tend to be more respectful of our physical body and its needs. I literally cannot believe that this is the same body that went to 3 day raves twenty years ago.

More Time for Self-Care: We often become better at prioritising self-care. We know that taking care of ourselves is essential to allow us to keep going at the same pace and we are more willing to carve out time for activities that are good for our soul, like reading, meditating, or pursuing our favourite hobbies. What you need from self-care will probably be changing too. From your yoga practice to your skin care routine, your body is now different and needs different care, whether you like that or not.

Deeper Sense of Purpose: Women often report feeling a deeper sense of purpose and meaning in their lives in midlife. I definitely do. I spent most of my twenties being an insecure wreck and my thirties being a working wife and mother that rarely slept. Now, for the first time ever, I can honestly say that I am comfortable and confident in myself. Not as a mother or as a yoga teacher, but as ME. I know who I am and I know my priorities and understand my values and I am unlikely to stray far from those.

You're likely going to have more time to reflect on what is important, and you are more likely to focus on your passions and purpose-driven activities that bring you a sense of fulfilment. This is the time to do this!

Life after 40 comes with many incredible gifts. As we celebrate the beauty and power that come with age and experience, we can inspire and uplift other women to do the same. This isn't just positive 'fluff.' Take a moment to really let this stuff sink in. Let us continue to support and empower each other as we move through this journey, knowing that the best is yet to come.

13. Embracing the 'Enchantress' and 'Wise Woman' Phases of Life

I'm fascinated by the power of embodying the qualities of the goddess archetypes. We can look at how these archetypes resonate through the different life stages and their appearance in the changing phases of the menstrual and lunar cycles. Understanding each of the archetypes and why they are relevant to us at every life stage, can help us identify what's happening within ourselves and also to focus on the positives of ageing. Let's explore how and when we may be drawn to embody each of Goddesses. I honestly can't think of a better time to do this than when going through the massive life translation that is perimenopause.

I mentioned the Maiden and Mother archetypes earlier and how they haven't always been used in a positive way to define female roles. This is not an entirely fair representation, as each of the goddess archetypes is strong, powerful, and multifaceted. But really, what comes next? What's after motherhood? Or what if you never choose to be or were able to become a mother?

We briefly touched upon the decimation of the Crone archetype throughout history and as we move into this new chapter, I invite you to meet the Enchantress (wild woman) and dive deeper into the Crone (wise woman) archetype and explore how we can embody their strengths during these transitions.

The Enchantress

The enchantress or wild woman archetype is an extremely powerful and positive force for us as we transition past the maiden and mother phases. She represents a woman who is in touch with her wild, primal and sensual nature. She is confident, passionate and unapologetically herself. This is so true of where many of us are in life as our children get older, or we move into new roles in our careers, and we get to embrace our true selves in a way that we never had the time or wisdom to do before.

The enchantress archetype has roots in many different cultures and traditions, from Greek mythology to Native American and Celtic traditions. In these cultures, the wild woman was often seen as a symbol of untamed nature, sensuality and fertility. She is often depicted as a seductress, a healer, a warrior or a goddess, depending on the culture and context. In many traditions, she represents the untamed and raw aspects of femininity, as well as the transformative power of the feminine life force. She was someone who was in touch with the natural world, and her

Embracing the 'Enchantress' and 'Wise Woman' Phases of Life

natural cycles are deeply attuned with the greater universe.

In more recent times, the wild woman archetype has been embraced as a symbol of the divine feminine, female empowerment and self-discovery. This archetype represents a force that we can tap into as we age, allowing us to embrace our own sensuality, passion and creativity, things sadly neglected in favour of caring for partners, careers and children.

One of the reasons why this archetype is so incredible is because it offers a fresh perspective on a woman's sexuality and sensuality. In our culture, women's sexuality has been repressed and marginalised for centuries, with an emphasis on modesty and purity and with many religions suppressing the very concept of women even having a right to sexuality. But the wild woman archetype challenges this view and shows that our sexuality can be empowering and transformative. By welcoming our sensual nature, we can tap into our feminine instincts and intuition and become a confident and passionate force for change in our own lives and in the world around us.

The enchantress archetype is particularly relevant as our children begin to leave home, and we get time to 'be ourselves' again. By welcoming enchantress or wild woman energy into our lives, we are initiating sexual discovery and exploration, on our own or with a partner. By owning our sexuality, it helps to increase our self-confidence and in our ability to love and look after ourselves.

Embody the Enchantress

The best way to embrace the enchantress is to explore your sensuality and sexuality. This could involve uncovering your desires and passions and finding ways to express them not just through erotic contact but through movement, art or dance. For example, you might take up a new hobby like burlesque dancing, life drawing or erotic writing and use these activities to tap into your own instinctive sensual nature. You might also explore your body through self-pleasure, using a yoni egg or sensual massage and allow yourself to experience pleasure in your own skin. This is not to be neglected and self-pleasure is just as important than sex with a partner. It helps us to love and connect with our own bodies and to understand our sexual needs.

Another way to embody the wild woman is to connect with the natural world. This could be as simple as spending more time in nature, literally hugging some trees or exploring your own primal and wild nature. For example, you might go for a long hike in the woods, go glamping with friends or spend an afternoon by the ocean and allow yourself to connect with the rhythms and cycles of the ocean and the natural world. You might want to explore your own connection to the elements and find ways to honour and celebrate them through ritual or meditation.

Another way to embody the enchantress is to connect with other women who are at the same stage of life and going through similar experiences. Nothing is more important now than connection. This could be joining a women's circle or group and sharing wisdom and support. You might also explore your ancestral or cultural roots and find ways to connect with the traditions and practices of your ancestors. I recently mapped out my family tree and found that I've descended from King James IV of Scotland on one side of my family and mostly Irish gipsies on the other side, and I found it so interesting. So far, I've got as far back as the fourteenth century.

The enchantress has a deep sense of her own worth and inner knowing and her senses are highly attuned. She represents the more mystical parts of the female psyche and is highly evolved and strong in her sense of self. In terms of lunar phases, the wild woman archetype is often associated with the moon's waning or last quarter phase.

The Wild Woman, The Waning Moon, and Your Yoga Practice

In the menstrual cycle, the waning moon corresponds to the premenstrual phase, which is also characterised by heightened emotional sensitivity, intuitive abilities and creative expression. This is a transitional phase from outward to inward energy, and you may find you want to spend more time alone or playing with your tarot cards or crystals when the moon is waning, as you embrace this wild woman energy. This phase is traditionally associated with introspection, inner work and the release of old patterns and emotions. It's a time for turning inward, examining your shadows and cultivating self-awareness. It's the process of withdrawal before the arrival of the new moon and the wise woman phase.

This is also a time of release and letting go when the moon is moving from fullness to darkness. During the waning moon, we can tap into our own inner wisdom and let go of anything that no longer serves us. This is a time to release old patterns and beliefs and to create space for new growth and transformation. This is very much reflected in our perimenopausal life too.

The Wild Woman archetype celebrates the diversity and richness of the feminine experience, beyond the limited and often oppressive stereotypes imposed by patriarchal culture. She invites us to reclaim our innate power and to reconnect with our bodies, emotions and intuition.

To embody the Wild Woman in your yoga practice, you can focus on poses that cultivate strength, flexibility and fluidity, such as hip openers, backbends and inversions. You can also incorporate movements that are inspired by animals, such as cat-cow, lion's breath and downward dog, bringing in that universal connection.

Meditation and pranayama practices can also help you connect with the Wild Woman, by cultivating a sense of inner stillness and awareness. You can try focusing on your breath, repeating a mantra or affirmation or visualising yourself in a natural setting, such as a forest or a beach or try the meditation I've provided below.

Perimenopause is a time to celebrate our own wild and primal nature, and to embrace our own sensuality and passion, more so than ever before. Allow the wild woman to guide you.

Enchantress Yoga Practice

This yoga sequence can help to feel empowered, confident, and free as we experience shifts in our identity. Each pose is designed to strengthen the body, improve balance and stability, and promote feelings of expansion and vitality.

Cat-Cow Pose (Marjaryasana/Bitilasana)

Start on your hands and knees, with your wrists directly under your shoulders and your knees directly under your hips. Inhale and arch your spine, lifting your tailbone and head towards the sky (Cow Pose). Exhale and round your spine, bringing your chin towards your chest and tucking your tailbone under (Cat Pose). Repeat this flow for several breaths. Cat-curls help to stretch the spine and release tension in the back and neck. It also helps to improve flexibility and increase energy.

Goddess Pose (Uttkata Konasana)

From a standing position, step your feet out wide and turn your toes out to the sides. Bend your knees and lower your hips, coming into a squatting position with your thighs parallel to the ground. Bring your hands to your heart centre and press your elbows against your inner thighs. This helps to strengthen the legs, hips, and lower back. It also helps to improve balance and flexibility, while promoting feelings of empowerment and confidence.

Warrior III (Virabhadrasana III)

From a standing position, shift your weight onto your right foot and lift your left leg behind you, parallel to the ground. Extend your arms out in front of you, reaching forward as you lift your leg higher. Keep your hips squared towards the ground and your gaze forward. This pose helps to improve balance and stability, while strengthening the legs, core, and back muscles. It also helps to promote feelings of strength and courage.

Half Moon Pose (Ardha Chandrasana)

From Warrior III, lower your left foot to the ground and straighten your right leg. Reach your right hand down towards the ground, placing it on a block or the floor.

Lift your left leg behind you, coming into a half-moon shape with your body. Reach your left arm up towards the sky. Half-moon pose helps to improve balance and stability, while strengthening the legs and core muscles. It also helps to stretch the hips, hamstrings, and side body, promoting feelings of expansiveness and freedom.

Tree Pose (Vrrkasana)

From a standing position, shift your weight onto your left foot and lift your right foot off the ground. Place the sole of your right foot against your inner left thigh or calf and bring your hands to your heart centre. Keep your gaze forward and your breath steady. Tree pose helps to improve balance and stability, while strengthening the legs and core muscles. It also helps to promote feelings of groundedness and connection to the earth.

Goddess Victory Pose (Urdhva Dhanurasana)

Lie on your back with your knees bent and your feet hip-distance apart. Place your hands on the ground next to your ears, with your fingertips pointing towards your shoulders. Inhale and press into your hands and feet, lifting your hips and chest towards the sky. Keep your elbows parallel to each other and your gaze towards the sky. This pose helps to stretch the entire body, including the chest, back, arms, and legs. It also helps to improve strength and flexibility, while promoting feelings of victory and success.

Enchantress meditation practice

This is a simple but effective meditation you can use at any time, but perhaps you are called to it when you are premenstrual or during the waning moon phase especially. You can embody the wild woman energy at any time and this meditation will offer you focus. Meditation can be a powerful tool for women seeking to connect with their inner enchantress.

By embracing the energy of the wild woman, we can tap into our sensual power and find new ways to express our desires and passions. Whether through meditation or other spiritual practices, by harnessing the energy of the enchantress, we can begin to transform our lives and become the wild and free-spirited women we were always meant to be. Yeeha!

How to do it:

To begin, find a quiet and comfortable space where you can sit or lie down comfortably. Close your eyes, and take a few deep breaths, allowing yourself to relax and release any tension or stress.

Once you feel centred and calm, begin to visualise yourself as the enchantress archetype. See yourself as a powerful and free-spirited woman, connected to the natural world and to your own inner wisdom and intuition. Allow yourself to feel the energy of the enchantress flowing through you and embrace the feeling of freedom and creativity that comes with it.

Embracing the 'Enchantress' and 'Wise Woman' Phases of Life

As you continue to visualise yourself as the enchantress, begin to focus on your breath. Take deep, slow breaths, inhaling through your nose and exhaling through your mouth. As you inhale, imagine yourself drawing in the energy of the earth and the cosmos, and as you exhale, imagine yourself releasing any tension or negativity.

Now, bring your awareness to your body. Notice any sensations or feelings that arise and allow yourself to fully experience them without judgement. If you feel any discomfort or tension, imagine yourself sending love and healing energy to those areas.

As you continue to breathe deeply and connect with your body, begin to focus on your desires and passions. What do you want to create in your life? What brings you joy and fulfilment? Allow yourself to fully embrace your desires and passions and see them as a natural and powerful expression of your enchantress energy.

Finally, when you feel ready, slowly bring yourself back to the present moment. Take a few deep breaths and open your eyes. Take a moment to reflect on your experience and consider how you can bring the energy of the enchantress into your daily life.

The Wise Woman

As we move through and past menopause, we enter what is known as the 'wise woman' phase of life. This is a time when we can draw upon all those juicy life experiences, knowledge and honed intuition to guide us forward. Embracing this phase of life and seeing it as an opportunity for growth and self-discovery is going to keep you focused, positive and strong.

In many cultures, the 'wise woman' or 'crone' archetype represents a powerful, regenerating force that we can view as a kind of 'rebirth'. This is particularly relevant as we move past menopause, as it is a time of transition and change that can be challenging but also very transformative.

Like the Enchantress, the wise woman archetype has roots in different cultures and philosophies across the globe, from Wicca to ancient Indian philosophy and Shamanic traditions. In these cultures, the wise woman was often seen as a healer, teacher and spiritual guide. She was someone who had lived a long and full life and who had gained wisdom and knowledge through her experiences. She was respected and revered and seen as a valued member of the community—very different from how women at a certain age are generally seen in popular culture today.

In more recent times, women, feminists, and spiritual seekers are embracing the wise woman as a symbol of empowerment as we move past our fertile years. This is the most powerful of the goddess archetypes and allows us to really draw upon our life experiences

Embracing the 'Enchantress' and 'Wise Woman' Phases of Life

and inner wisdom to help guide us through life's challenges.

One of the reasons why the wise woman archetype is so incredible is because she offers a positive perspective on getting older. The wise woman challenges the view that ageing is a bad thing and shows that it can be a rejuvenating and empowering experience for women.

A simple way to embody the wise woman or crone is to really embrace your own wisdom and life experiences—good and bad. Reflect on your life, the loves, the opportunities that you had and missed and what you learned from each. This reflection on your own life journey and recognizing the lessons and insights you have gained along the way, can be powerful in itself. For example, you might journal about your experiences or meditate on the lessons you have learned. You may also want to share your wisdom and experience with others and mentor or support younger women or family members who are going through transitions or similar experiences.

Another way to embody the wise woman is to connect with the cycles of life and death. This can involve honouring and celebrating the natural cycles of birth, growth, decay and death. For example, you might create a sacred space or altar at home or in your garden to honour the changing seasons, or you might participate in rituals or ceremonies that celebrate the transitions of life.

Just as with the Enchantress archetype, a great way to fully embrace the wise woman is to connect with other women who are going through this transition too: Sharing wisdom and supporting other women who are also navigating life post-menopause. You may also want to seek out the guidance and wisdom of other wise women in your life, such as elders or spiritual leaders.

The Crone, The New Moon and Yoga

In terms of lunar phases, the crone archetype is often associated with the new moon. At this time of the month, the archetypal wise woman steps forward. This is the Crone Goddess, *'She who sees everything'*. The wise woman helps you to refine your power by taking your awareness deep within for intuitive insight and leaving a legacy of wisdom for other women to follow.

The wise woman archetype is positive because it represents a time of life when we can let go of societal expectations and focus on our own needs and desires. It is a time for introspection and the pursuit of your deepest passions. - the things you never did but always wanted to. As a woman in the Crone phase of life you have the opportunity to become a leader and role model, passing down your learned experiences and wisdom to future generations.

In terms of your yoga practice, the Crone archetype is associated with slow and reflective practices, such as restorative yoga, yin yoga and Yoga Nidra. These practices help women to connect deeply with their feminine intuition and to cultivate self-awareness. If you've neglected to connect with your physical body and true self, now is the time to do that. The Crone phase is also a time to focus on physically strengthening the bones and joints, as well as improving your balance and stability.

During the new moon, we should practise yoga poses that promote introspection, such as forward folds and twists. These poses help us to find calm in the storm of the menopausal mind and create a sense of deep peace and contentment. The Crone phase is also a time to really focus on pranayama and meditation, which can help us to reduce stress, and anxiety and promote an overall sense of inner strength.

Welcoming The Wise Woman Yoga Practice

This sequence will help you embrace your inner wisdom, groundedness, and feminine strength. Each pose is designed to help you de-stress, improve your balance and stability, and promote healthy digestion and elimination. Practicing this sequence regularly can help you feel more confident, empowered, and at peace.

Easy Pose (Sukkhasana)

Sit cross-legged on your mat with your hands resting on your knees. Close your eyes and take several deep breaths, focusing on your breath and bringing your awareness inward. Easy pose helps to calm you down and increases feelings of relaxation.

Seated Twist (Ardha Matsyendrasana)

From Easy Pose, place your right hand on your left knee and your left hand behind your back. Inhale and lengthen your spine, then exhale and twist towards the left, using your right hand to deepen the twist. Hold for several breaths, then repeat on the other side. Twists help to stretch the spine and promote healthy digestion. It also helps to release tension in the back and shoulders, promoting feelings of relaxation and ease.

Downward Facing Dog (Adho Mukkha Svanasana)

Come onto your hands and knees, with your wrists directly under your shoulders and your knees directly under your hips. Exhale and lift your hips up towards the sky, coming into an inverted V shape. Press your hands and feet firmly into the ground, and let your head hang down between your arms. Down dog helps to stretch the entire body, including the back, hamstrings, and shoulders. It also helps to strengthen the arms and legs, while promoting feelings of grounding.

Garland Pose (Malasana)

From Downward Facing Dog, step your feet forward to the front of your mat and lower your hips down into a squatting position. Bring your hands together in front of your heart and press your elbows against your inner thighs. This pose helps to stretch the hips, groin, and lower back. It also helps to improve digestion and promote healthy elimination, while promoting feelings of inner strength and stability.

Tree Pose (Vrrkasana)

From a standing position, shift your weight onto your left foot and lift your right foot off the ground. Place the sole of your right foot against your inner left thigh or calf and bring your hands to your heart centre. Keep your gaze forward and your breath steady. Tree pose helps balance and stability, while strengthening the legs and core muscles. It also helps with connection to the earth.

Corpse Pose (Savasana)

Lie down on your back with your legs extended and your arms at your sides. Close your eyes and allow your body to fully relax, releasing any tension or stress. Stay in this pose for several minutes, focusing on your breath and letting go of any thoughts or worries. Corpse helps you to relax and restore the body and mind. It helps to reduce stress and anxiety.

Wise Woman Meditation

This is a meditation practice that can help you connect with your deepest wise woman. The crone is associated with qualities like wisdom, experience and spiritual insight. When you embody this archetype in meditation, you can cultivate a deeper sense of self-awareness and acceptance. This can help you to let go of any self-judgement or doubt that may arise during menopause and approach this phase of life with greater confidence and ease.

How To Do It:

To begin, find a quiet and comfortable space where you can sit or lie down comfortably. Close your eyes, and take a few deep breaths, allowing yourself to relax and release any tension or stress.

Once you feel centred and calm, begin to visualise yourself as the wise woman or crone archetype. See yourself as a woman who is wise, powerful and full of knowledge and experience. Imagine yourself surrounded by a circle of otherwise women, who are there to support you and share their wisdom with you.

As you continue to visualise yourself as the wise woman or crone, begin to focus on your breath. Take deep, slow breaths, inhaling through your nose and exhaling through your mouth. As you inhale, imagine yourself drawing in the energy of the earth and the cosmos, and as you exhale, imagine yourself releasing any tension or negativity.

Embracing the 'Enchantress' and 'Wise Woman' Phases of Life

Now, bring your awareness to your body. Notice any sensations or feelings that arise and allow yourself to fully experience them without judgement. If you feel any discomfort or tension, imagine yourself sending love and healing energy to those areas.

As you continue to breathe deeply and connect with your body, begin to focus on the wisdom and experience that you have gained in your life. Think about the challenges that you have faced and the lessons that you have learned. Allow yourself to feel a sense of gratitude for all that you have experienced and for the person that you have become.

Finally, when you feel ready, slowly bring yourself back to the present moment. Take a few deep breaths and open your eyes. Take a moment to reflect on your experience and consider how you can bring the wisdom and grace of the wise woman or crone into your daily life.

Through regular meditation practice, you can cultivate a deeper sense of self-compassion and inner strength, which can help you to weather the challenges of menopause with greater ease.

14. Strategies for overcoming challenges and sticking to your wellness practices

Committing to the appropriate wellness rituals and practices on both the good days and the bad, is essential for managing your symptoms and staying positive. In this chapter, we'll discuss some strategies for understanding your triggers, overcoming challenges that we didn't see coming, and remembering why you created your wellness goals through the rough and the smooth.

Identify Your Triggers

The first step to making sure that you stick to your wellness practices, is identifying and understanding your triggers. This includes anything that might trigger symptoms, things like hot flashes, mood swings or overwhelming fatigue. Once you know what those triggers are, you can develop a plan for managing them. For example, if you know that stress triggers your hot flashes, you can develop a mini plan for reducing stress, such as a specific asana or meditation.

Develop a Routine

Set aside time each day for self-care practices, such as your yoga practice, a walking meditation in nature or journaling. Having a consistent routine can also help regulate your sleep patterns, which is important for managing symptoms. Check out the suggested daily routine I provided earlier and consider what your personal routine might look like throughout the month.

Find a Support System

Find friends or family members who understand what you're going through and can give you unconditional support and encouragement. Joining a women's yoga or support group or online community can also be helpful. You can join my free Facebook community here, there are a gorgeous group of women from across the world who are there to support you on your journey and have a few laughs along the way.

Make Small Changes

Making minor changes can be easier than trying to make a load of big changes all at once. Start by making one small change at a time, like adding more vegetables to your diet, practising mindful eating or taking a short walk every day. Once you've mastered one mini-change, add another one! Over time, these slight changes can add up to big improvements in your overall health and well-being. Making these little daily changes is the basis of my Yoga Life Detox, where I help women transform their lives with just a tiny bit of time and effort each day. Do not estimate the power of the little things: Those tiny factors make up your larger life.

Focus on Mindful Eating and Good Nutrition

Please don't ignore this one! As a woman who is often a sucker for a Cosmo and a Curry—this has been a big deal for me. At 43, I can no longer eat anything I want and look and feel the way I used to: You just cannot ignore this! Nutrition is also a crucial aspect of managing perimenopause symptoms. Eating a balanced diet needs to include plenty of fruits and vegetables, lean protein and whole grains can help with managing symptoms such as hot flashes, fatigue and mood swings. Avoiding alcohol, caffeine and spicy foods can also really help manage symptoms, even though you may not want to hear this.

Prioritise Movement

Aim for at least 30 minutes of exercise every day, simple activities like walking, yoga or swimming. If you're not used to exercising, start slowly and gradually build up your activity level.

Get Enough Sleep

Sleep is crucial for managing perimenopause symptoms and staying active. Aim for 7–8 hours of sleep per night—8–10 if you can get it—and establish a consistent sleep routine. Avoid using your phone or other electronic devices before bedtime, as the blue light can interfere with your sleep.

Remember to listen to your body and seek professional help when needed. You've got this!

Pause for Thought ...

Finding the support and resources that you need during perimenopause

This book is a great start, but there are tons of different types of support and resources available out there, and it's important to find the ones that work best for you. Where this book focuses mostly on yoga and meditation, there are a lot of other aspects of the menopause journey that you probably want to investigate. You may also want to consider my online perimenopause programme, *The YogaPause*, which goes in depth into every aspect of embracing this life stage.

Here are a couple of ideas around support and making connections right now:

Connect with other women: One of the best things you can do for yourself is to connect with other women who are going through the same thing. Connecting with others can help you feel less alone and provide you with those valuable information and resources.

Find a healthcare provider who listens: It's important to have a physician or practitioner who listens to your concerns and takes them seriously. If you don't feel like your current provider is meeting your needs, don't be afraid to look for someone else who can better support you. I've been there and been fobbed off with the 'all women have to go through it.' You don't. There are options and solutions.

Make sure you have a yoga teacher who understands perimenopause and how to not only adapt your practice but can provide a practice created for this life stage. Honestly, look no further than my YogaPause teachers.

Explore holistic therapies: In addition to traditional medical treatments, there are many natural therapies that can be beneficial during perimenopause. From acupuncture to herbal remedies, there are a variety of options available to help support you.

Practice self-care: If it's not been a big part of your life before due to a lack of time or other commitments, now is the time to make time for things that keep you balanced and motivated. This could be anything from taking a relaxing bath, to crochet, to practising yoga or meditation. Whatever floats your boat, do that.

Stay informed: Knowledge is power, and the more you know about the menopause journey and its impact on your body and mind, the better equipped you will be to manage its challenges. Stay informed by reading books, attending workshops or webinars and talking to your healthcare provider.

Get professional help: If you are struggling with depression, anxiety or other mental health issues, don't hesitate to seek professional help. There is no shame in this and it's something that many women go through.

Pause for Thought ...

A mental health professional can provide you with the support and resources.

15. Superfoods, Eating and The Right Nutrition for Optimal Health and Longevity

Understanding the role of nutrition in staying fit and frisky

An important (and often conveniently overlooked) factor that plays a significant role in managing perimenopause well, is nutrition. In this chapter, we'll look at optimal nutrition in perimenopause, including how specific nutrients and dietary choices can help manage your symptoms and support vitality.

The hormonal changes that affect our metabolism, energy levels and mood, also result in making our bodies more sensitive to certain foods and we may need to make some changes to what we consume. As always, it's important to listen to your body and make food choices that work for you, rather than following a one-size-fits-all approach or being focused on 'fad diets' and weight loss.

That said, one of the main nutritional concerns for women throughout menopause is maintaining a healthy weight. As we get older, our bodies become less efficient at metabolising glucose, which can lead to weight gain and an increased risk of developing chronic diseases, like type 2 diabetes. To maintain a healthy weight, we need a well-rounded diet that includes nutrient-rich foods, like leafy greens, whole grains, lean proteins and healthy fats. Additionally, portion control and avoiding excessive added sugars and saturated fats can really help regulate our weight and keep us feeling fabulous.

Another important nutritional consideration to keep in mind is that eating the right food can help with managing hot flashes and night sweats. These can also be made worse by some foods and drinks, including things like caffeine, alcohol and spicy foods. To minimise these symptoms, look at reducing their intake as they are big triggers and instead try to incorporate foods that are rich in phytoestrogens, such as soy, flaxseeds and chickpeas. Phytoestrogens are plant-based compounds that have a mild oestrogen-like effect and may help to reduce the incidence and frequency of both.

Bone health is also a big consideration, as we are now at an increased risk of osteoporosis and fractures. To help support bone health, we should aim to eat foods rich in calcium and vitamin D, which are both essential for building and maintaining strong bones. Good sources of calcium include things like dairy products, leafy greens, almonds and fortified foods such as orange juice. You can get your dose of Vitamin D from sun exposure, fatty fish and fortified dairy products too.

Hormonal mood swings, anxiety and depression are also affected by our diet. While there is no single 'mood-boosting' food, eating nutrient-dense foods, fresh fruits and vegetables, whole grains and lean proteins can help support your overall well-being. Additionally, incorporating foods that are high in mood-boosting nutrients, such as omega-3 fatty acids and magnesium, can also help. Good sources of omega-3 fatty acids include foods like fatty fish, flaxseeds and walnuts while magnesium-rich foods include leafy greens, nuts and whole grains.

Hormone-Happy Recommendations for a Balanced Diet

Here is a quick 'cheat sheet' of recommendations to help you create a nutritious and well-rounded diet during perimenopause:

1. **Focus on whole, nutrient-dense foods:** Aim to eat mostly whole, minimally processed foods that are rich in nutrients. Things such as fruits, vegetables, whole grains and lean proteins. These will provide you with the vitamins, minerals and antioxidants your body needs.

2. **Get enough protein:** It's essential for maintaining healthy muscles, bones and skin, as well as supporting a healthy immune system. Aim to include lean protein sources like chicken, fish, tofu and legumes into your diet.

3. **Include healthy fats:** Fats are an important part of a healthy diet and can help you feel full and satisfied. Opt for healthy fats such as avocados, olive oil, nuts and seeds, and limit your intake of unhealthy fats such as trans fats and saturated fats.

4. **Limit sugar and refined carbohydrates:** High sugar and refined carbohydrate intake can increase insulin levels, which can contribute to weight gain and other health problems. Try to limit your intake of sugar and refined carbohydrates and opt for complex carbohydrates such as whole grains instead.

5. **Stay hydrated:** I don't need to say it again. Lots of water can help manage symptoms like hot flashes and mood swings. Aim to drink at least 8 glasses of water per day and limit your intake of sugary drinks such as coke and juices.

6. **Include calcium-rich foods:** This is essential for maintaining strong bones. Including calcium-rich foods such as dairy products, leafy greens and fortified foods are just perfect.

Pause for Thought ...

7. **Get enough vitamins and minerals:** Also essential for overall health and managing symptoms like fatigue and hormonal mood swings. Make sure you eat a variety of nutrient-rich foods and consider taking a multivitamin supplement (check out my recommended herbs and supplements shortly).

Want more specifics? You can check out some of my tasty perimenopause-friendly recipes at the back of the book too.

Eat, Binge and Avoid

There are certain foods that can help support you throughout menopause while others will make things much worse. Let's look in a bit more depth at what to eat and avoid.

Certain foods can help balance your hormone levels even while your body is going through all these tempestuous, mind-boggling changes. It doesn't mean they will stop perimenopause from happening, but they may help make this phase a little more palatable. I'm diving a bit deeper into what's good and what's got to go from your plate.

GO FOR THESE:

Calcium and Vitamin D-rich foods. Foods like kale, turnips, seaweed, milk and collards. Vitamin D can be found in cod liver oil, tuna, yoghurt, eggs and salmon.

Vegetables, especially leafy greens like kale, Swiss chard, collard greens, arugula and bok choy. Vegetable intake is great for weight loss during perimenopause as it's normal to gain some extra weight due to hormonal changes.

- **Cruciferous and sulphur-rich vegetables** such as brussels sprouts, kale, spinach and asparagus help the body make Diindolylmethane. Diindolylmethane, or DIM for short, helps in the balancing of the body's hormones by aiding in the breakdown of oestrogen. The breakdown of excess oestrogen is a necessity if the end goal is overall hormonal balance in the body.

- **High-fibre foods** include lentils, black beans, peas, broccoli, raspberries, pears and oatmeal. Fibre will help with your digestive health and weight control too and help you feel full longer.

Berries are full of fibre and packed with antioxidants. They contain less sugar than most fruits, helping curb your sugar cravings.

Protein helps you feel fuller, making it less likely to snack between meals. Protein will help reduce hunger, helps curb cravings and also protects muscle mass. Include eggs, lean meats, fish, nuts and seeds, tofu, tempeh, edamame and soy milk. When consuming tofu, always make sure you are leaning toward organic brands.

Pause for Thought ...

Legumes are also high in protein and fibre, which will help you feel full, which is very helpful when battling perimenopause weight gain. They can help stabilise blood sugar levels and decrease mood swings. Legumes to include in your diet include peas, beans, and lentils.

Phytoestrogen-rich foods: Phytoestrogens are found in whole foods. They do not cause oestrogen excess like xenoestrogens in the environment do. Studies show isoflavones may act as antioestrogens protecting women from stronger oestrogens such as oestradiol. Phytoestrogens down-regulate the activity of some oestrogen receptors prominent in breast and uterine tissue. This is one possible action behind their projected anticancer effects. Flax seeds and other seeds, legumes, grains and vegetables such as yams, carrots and apples have phytoestrogens.

Probiotic-rich foods or Cultured foods help keep your gut microbiome thriving. Research is emerging demonstrating a connection between the gut microbiome and hormone balance. Researchers now believe that certain microbes in the gut secrete and modulate hormones to such an extent that the gut microbiota should be classified as part of the endocrine system!

To cultivate a robust gut microbiome, incorporate cultured foods such as cultured vegetables, sauerkraut, beet kvass, sugar-free non-dairy yoghurt, kombucha and water kefir.

Another easy way to strengthen your microbiome is to feed it! One of my favourite tips is to make a Microbiome Mash. This mash is a mix of as many varieties of veggies as possible to feed gut bacteria. The easiest way to do this is to put various vegetables and greens and pulse in a food processor until everything is pretty small (and more easily digestible). Begin by adding 1–2 tablespoons of your microbiome mash to your meals daily—depending on the variety of veg and greens you choose—you may enjoy sautéing your mash a little and adding it to cooked foods or try a small amount in a smoothie! Watch this video for more on how to create a **Microbiome Veggie Mash—** https://www.youtube.com/watch?v=ImHQAvY6Wu8&t=19s

Seeds are the perfect hormone food! Seeds have ligands that bind excess hormones so they can be removed from the body. As well, they are high in omega-3 fats which help with hormone production. A super combo! I love hemp, chia and flax to keep my hormones in check.

Wild-caught, low-mercury seafood. Seafood supports healthy iodine levels, vitamin D levels, testosterone levels and much more! Choose low-mercury seafood like shrimp, scallops, clams, oysters, salmon, and sardines. **Fatty fish** is known to decrease inflammation, reduce night sweats, improve mood and help with depression. Some fatty fish include salmon, sardines and tuna.

Zinc-rich foods help boost testosterone and support immune function. Testosterone levels decline as we move toward menopause. Studies have shown that a decrease in testosterone is a common reason for reduced libido in perimenopausal women. Foods that are high in magnesium, such as hemp seeds, spinach and figs, increase testosterone. Maple syrup, cocoa powder and any chocolate product that is at least 40% cocoa, sunflower seeds, pine nuts, pumpkin, most nuts and most cuts of beef and lamb generally have 4 mg zinc per 100-gram serving. 2–3 servings daily with your meals can meet your need for zinc.

Superfoods

We've talked about good foods for perimenopause, but how about superfoods? Everyone's raving about 'Superfoods', and they make it into this category because they are nutrient-dense and typically have qualities that are more beneficial per bite than other foods.

Below are some of the superfoods that you want to be feasting on right now:

- Reishi supports the endocrine and immune systems as well as supports a healthy stress response

- Chaga, an adaptogen that helps manage stress and supports the immune system

- Bee pollen provides an energy boost, reduces the amount of stress the body is under safely and naturally and may help manage irritability, depression, immune deficiency and anxiety

- Coconut oil: this medium-chain fat has antibacterial and antifungal properties. It can help support healthy brain and gut function and is an alternative moisturiser and lubricant (do not use latex condoms).

- Sea vegetables provide much-needed iodine for the thyroid gland, breast tissue and energy production. You can add kelp sprinkles to food, add spirulina to smoothies or take chlorella tablets. If you have any issues with sodium, you may need to lower your sea veggie intake.

Now, let's talk about the foods to avoid

While it's important to focus on getting a lot of those whole, nutrient-dense foods, there are certain foods that can exacerbate symptoms during perimenopause. Some of the foods to avoid or limit include:

- Processed foods: Processed foods like fast food, candy and snack cakes can contribute to inflammation in the body, which can exacerbate symptoms.

- Sugar: Excessive sugar consumption can also contribute to inflammation, as well as insulin resistance, which can affect hormone balance.

- Caffeine: While some women can tolerate caffeine just fine; others find that it exacerbates symptoms like hot flashes and anxiety.

- Alcohol: Excessive alcohol consumption can affect sleep quality and contribute to inflammation, so it's important to drink in moderation or avoid alcohol altogether.

By paying attention to what you eat and making a conscious effort to focus on whole, nutrient-dense foods, you can support your health and well-being during perimenopause.

Understanding food sensitivities and allergies and how they could impact your health.

I mentioned earlier that our bodies may begin to respond differently to different types of food as we get older. Firstly, let's differentiate between food sensitivities and allergies. A food allergy is a reaction of the immune system to a particular food protein, which can range from mild symptoms like hives to severe, life-threatening reactions like anaphylaxis. In contrast, food sensitivities do not involve the immune system but rather the digestive system's inability to break down certain foods. Symptoms of food sensitivities include joys such as excessive bloating, diarrhoea, constipation and abdominal pain.

Perimenopause can often bring about quite dramatic changes in digestive health and food tolerance. Hormonal fluctuations often impact our digestive system's ability to break down and absorb certain foods, leading to new or heightened sensitivities and allergies.

So, how can food sensitivities and allergies impact our overall wellness during perimenopause? Here are some ways you may see this:

Hormonal imbalances: Certain food sensitivities and allergies can trigger further hormonal imbalances and exacerbate symptoms such as hot flashes, mood swings and insomnia.

Inflammation: Food sensitivities and allergies can cause inflammation, leading to joint pain, skin rashes and gastrointestinal discomfort.

Nutrient deficiencies: Avoiding certain foods due to allergies or sensitivities can lead to nutrient deficiencies, which can impact overall health. If you must cut something out, make sure that it's supplemented in other ways.

Weight gain: Food sensitivities and allergies can lead to weight gain due to inflammation and digestive issues.

Pause for Thought ...

This is a basic overview of how food sensitivities and allergies can impact you as we get older, but it's important to understand some basic ways to manage them:

- **Keep a food diary:** Keep track of what you eat and any symptoms that arise. This can help identify trigger foods and help with managing symptoms.

- **Seek professional help:** Consult with a registered dietitian, naturopath or allergist to help identify and manage food sensitivities and allergies.

- **Try an elimination diet:** Eliminating common trigger foods like dairy, gluten, soy and corn for a set period and then reintroducing them can help identify food sensitivities and allergies.

- **Incorporate nutrient-dense foods:** Focus on incorporating nutrient-dense foods such as leafy greens, whole grains and lean protein to ensure you are getting enough nutrients.

- **Manage stress:** High-stress levels can exacerbate food sensitivities and allergies, so finding ways to manage stress, such as meditation or yoga, can help reduce symptoms.

There are a few food allergies that are more common in women over forty. Here are some of the main culprits:

Dairy: Dairy products contain lactose, which can be difficult for some people to digest, leading to bloating, abdominal pain and diarrhoea. As we age, our bodies produce less lactase, the enzyme responsible for breaking down lactose, which can trigger dairy allergies in perimenopausal women.

Gluten: Gluten is a protein found in wheat, barley and rye. Gluten sensitivity or intolerance can cause symptoms such as bloating, abdominal pain, diarrhoea and fatigue. Perimenopausal women may experience new or heightened gluten allergies due to hormonal changes impacting the digestive system's ability to break down gluten.

Soy: Soy products are a common allergen that can cause digestive issues, skin rashes and respiratory symptoms. Soy contains phytoestrogens, which mimic the effects of oestrogen in the body. Perimenopausal women with hormone imbalances may experience soy allergies due to an excess of oestrogen in the body.

Corn: Corn is a common allergen that can cause digestive issues, skin rashes and respiratory symptoms. Corn is also a common ingredient in processed foods, making it difficult to avoid. Perimenopausal women with hormonal imbalances may experience corn allergies due to the digestive system's inability to break down corn proteins.

Eggs: Eggs are a common allergen that can cause digestive issues, skin rashes and respiratory symptoms. Perimenopausal women may experience egg allergies due to hormonal imbalances impacting the immune system's response to egg proteins.

It's important to note that these are just a few examples of the many food allergies that can pop up during perimenopause. Each woman is unique, and food allergies can vary widely in type and severity. Keep an eye out for things like Shellfish allergies too.

The Best Herbs, Supplements, and Minerals for the Menopause Journey

'Added extras' like herbs and supplements can be great for easing symptoms, so I'm providing you with some of the best supplements that can support you as you go through this phase. Please check with your physician before taking any new supplements, especially if you are already on other medications.

Black cohosh:

- Actaea racemosa, a North American perennial herb widely used for the relief of menopausal symptoms including mood, muscle stiffness, joint pain and sleep disturbances

- Potential contraindications in people with breast cancer.
- Consider a tincture form of this herb so you can start with 1–2 drops. Only increase if needed and never use more than the recommended dose on the label.

DIM

- DIM (diindolylmethane) can help support balanced oestrogen levels and be especially beneficial for people struggling with fibrocystic breasts, uterine fibroids, endometriosis and severe PMS.
- The easiest way to include DIM in your plan is by eating up to a cup of radish sprouts daily. Make them yourself by placing 1 Tablespoon of radish seeds in 2 cups of cool water. Allow the seeds to soak overnight. Drain and rinse the seeds. Place the seeds in a clean mason jar and cover the opening with a piece of clean cloth secured with an elastic band so air can flow into the jar while bugs are kept out. When the first leaves or sprouts emerge, rinse the seeds with cool water, drain and cover again. Do this daily until ready to eat. In a few days, you should have a mason jar or delicious, spicy sprouts!

Probiotics

- Probiotics: a healthy gut is essential for healthy hormones, as they help move excess oestrogen out of the body

- Culturelle Digestive Daily Probiotic Capsules contain L. rhamnosus GG, which may help support digestive health and ease bloating and diarrhoea. Additionally, it contains the prebiotic inulin to support the gut's microbiome.

- Garden of Life Vaginal Care formula has 50 billion CFUs and 38 different strains of probiotics, including L. acidophilus and Bifidobacterium. Each capsule also contains a blend of raw fruits and vegetables as prebiotics that Garden of Life says is to support the natural growth of healthy vaginal flora.

- The bottom line, pun intended, is that you need to be having regular bowel movements to remove excess hormones and metabolic waste from your body!

B Vitamin Complex

- B vitamins help adrenals respond to stress and produce hormones that are declining in ovaries

Vitamin D + K2

- Look for a liquid form of this that is oil-based. Vitamin D is fat-soluble. The combination with K2 helps ensure that calcium is not leached from your bones!

- Use caution if you have any bleeding or clotting issues.

- 1,000-5,000IU daily based on a serum blood test showing your Vitamin D level.

L-theanine

- This amino acid promotes a state of calmness and helps reduce stress.

- 100mg taken at the onset of feeling stressed or before bed can be helpful.

Melatonin

- May help improve sleep and brain health that often declines during perimenopause.

- Start with 1mg about 40 minutes before bed and only increase if needed.

Maca

- This adaptogenic herb native to Peru is renowned for its hormone-balancing properties.

- Add maca powder to smoothies, soups or stews. In Peru, maca is used to make porridge. Start with a small amount and work your way up until you feel results. Because maca can jumpstart energy and libido, working up can be more comfortable.

- Femmenessence is a clinically proven maca product for menopause/perimenopause. May boost energy, increase libido, manage symptoms like hot flashes and supports a healthy cortisol response

Oats

- Oat groats are nourishing and even though they may seem simple. They are renowned as a medicinal food/supplement.

- Oat milk can help ease fatigue. And the fibre from whole oats promotes good bowel movements which help release metabolic waste!

Omega-3 fatty acids:

- Offers cardiovascular protection that is not as apparent as oestrogen levels decline.

- Good sources include fatty fish and hemp seeds. A supplement in capsule or liquid form can be helpful.

Rehmannia:

- a root that helps with cooling and grounding; may provide healthy ageing benefits

- may help prevent osteoporosis

- supports blood sugar balance

Safety note: Do your research and visit a practitioner who is well-trained and certified in using herbs and supplements. If you are interested in Chinese herbs, see a Traditional Chinese Medicine (TCM) practitioner for all Chinese herbs.

Rhodiola

- This is an adaptogenic herb that supports adrenal function and empowers you to handle stress better.

- Rhodiola is astringent and may help with fatigue and weakness. Because it is slightly stimulating, use it earlier in the day.

- Find a tincture form so you can easily control the dose.

Shatavari

- Shatavari is wild asparagus. In Ayurveda, it is considered a female tonic. Traditionally it has been used to boost libido, tame hot flashes, curb night sweating and lessen brain fog. Shatavari also has immunomodulating, apoptogenic and anti-stress effects.

- Customarily Shatavari is mixed with a glass of warm milk and honey, but it can be mixed into a wide range of dishes, drinks and teas.

- You can purchase Shatavari powder on Amazon.

Pause for Thought ...

Luscious Essential Oil Blends

Essential oils are another fantastic holistic tool that I have always been a huge fan of. These can be used therapeutically in perimenopause to ease most discomforts. I also love to use aroma blends in my yoga practice, whether that's through diffusion or application (I'll take you through the options). You do want to make sure you are using reputable brands that are certified pure therapeutic grade for safety and quality purposes. These essential oils are perfect for perimenopause, and I've explained why:

- Frankincense supports brain health and reduces symptoms of depression and anxiety

- Clary Sage supports hormone balance when applied to wrists and behind ears and manages symptoms of perimenopause, including hot flashes

- Peppermint helps reduce hot flashes, osteoporosis, cravings and digestive issues and muscle & joint pain

- Marjoram may help reduce chronic stress, menstrual concerns, and high blood pressure that often comes along with oestrogen reduction

How to use these essential oils:

Massage 2–4 drops diluted in fractionated coconut oil and massage into the abdomen, lower back and shoulders as a good starting point.

Here's a lovely custom aroma blend that I love to use myself. Combining these oils keep cortisol levels stable while calming your body and mind and supporting your libido and can naturally support oestrogen levels:

4 drops clary sage essential oil

3 drops of geranium essential oil

3 drops of bergamot essential oil

2 drops of lavender essential oil

2 drops of frankincense essential oil

1 drop of ylang-ylang essential oil

1 drop of peppermint essential oil

Directions for blending

1. Fill a small glass bottle with a carrier oil of your choice, such as jojoba or sweet almond oil.
2. Add the essential oils in the recommended number of drops to the carrier oil.
3. Close the bottle and gently shake it to mix the oils together.

To use, try applying a small amount of the blend to your wrists, neck or temples. You can also pop it into a rollerball and roll the blend over ovaries and pulse points 2 to 3 times per day. You can also add a few drops to a diffuser or inhale the aroma directly from the bottle.

This blend includes several essential oils that are thought to be great for perimenopause symptoms. Clary sage is known to help balance hormones and reduce hot flashes while geranium may help with mood swings and anxiety. Bergamot is believed to have a calming effect, and lavender is known for its ability to promote relaxation and restful sleep. Frankincense is thought to have anti-inflammatory properties, and ylang-ylang may help with mood and emotional balance. Peppermint is also included for its cooling effect and ability to help with headaches and other discomforts associated with perimenopause. Basically, this is your ideal lady-over-40 blend.

16. Pause for Thought ...

As we come to the end of this book ladies, I hope that you've gained a deeper understanding of what the menopause journey looks like and feel confident about the impact that the right yoga practice, good lifestyle choices, nutrition and the lovely PAM can have on your experience. Just being aware of these key pillars of health, you're already halfway to a vibrant, fruitful and frisky future.

We've explored how yoga can help to not only manage your hormonal symptoms, but also helps with things like keeping steady and focused on your resolve and life purpose. By incorporating all of the elements of the YogaPause Sadhana into your yoga practice, your practice will bring you so much more than just physical benefits. Things like increasing your strength, stamina, balance and bone density are just the tip of the iceberg when it comes to the bounties of yoga.

We've also looked at the importance of proper nutrition alongside the right movement, including the potential impact of food sensitivities and allergies on your health during perimenopause. By paying attention to what your body is telling you its needs and being aware of how it reacts to certain foods and food groups, you can increase your energy and look and feel better than ever before.

The most important factor in all of this, is the right mindset and your outlook on ageing. By embracing impermanence and understanding that ageing is not necessarily a bad thing or the demise of your value as a woman, you can look forward to many happy years of doing exactly what you want and what you never had the time to do before! Once you've grasped the value of the enchantress and wise woman, the world

Pause for Thought ...

becomes your oyster once again. We can tap into a new or renewed sense of inner strength and confidence and begin to really explore who we are outside of the shackles of motherhood or being someone's partner or other.

Most importantly, you are not alone. Community is vital for women at every life stage, but this is especially true now. Supporting other women, in turn, helps you to be supported through the community. Many studies even show that women who spend more quality time in the company of other women, live longer! Talk about what you are experiencing, about your personal remedies and challenges and how you've overcome them. When we don't want to admit or acknowledge that it's happening then we aren't openly discussing menopause, and we're perpetuating the idea that life ends at forty. Talk about growing older in the bright light that it deserves.

There are tons of resources and sources of support becoming available now, from specialist yoga teachers and nutritionists to mental health professionals and support groups. Each of these will help you feel empowered and confident, you just need to seek them out.

Remember that this is a time when we have immense potential for personal growth and transformation. By prioritising your own health and well-being (for once,) and actively cultivating a positive mindset, you can really live your best life and embrace all of the possibilities of this next stage. This phase of life has so much to offer, from being able to fully embrace your true self to newfound freedoms and opportunities. Be yourself; show yourself love and absolutely enjoy the ride ladies, because you have *everything* ahead of you.

17. Hormone-Balancing Recipes

Breakfast

Hormone Happy Latte

Serve 1

- 1 cup strongly brewed dandelion root tea
- 1 teaspoon maple syrup
- 1 teaspoon Shatavari powder
- 1 teaspoon maca powder
- ½ cup milk (dairy or dairy-free)

Instructions

1. Add all ingredients to a small pot on the stove over medium heat. Cook until steaming, but not boiling.
2. Pour into a mug and enjoy.

Heavens Eggs with Sesame

Serves 1

- 2 teaspoons coconut oil

- 3 eggs, whisked
- 2 tablespoons kimchi, chopped
- Sea salt and black pepper, to taste
- 1 toasted nori sheet, chopped into 1" squares
- 1 teaspoon toasted sesame seeds

Instructions

1. Add oil to a medium skillet over medium heat. When hot, stir in the eggs, kimchi, salt, and pepper.
2. Cook for 1 to 2 minutes or until eggs are cooked to your liking. Serve topped with nori and sesame seeds.

Superwoman Morning Cup

Serves 1

- 1 cup unsweetened yoghourt (dairy or dairy-free)
- 1 teaspoon chlorella powder
- 1 banana, sliced
- ¼ cup dried, unsulphured figs
- 1 tablespoon toasted pine nuts

- 1 pinch sea salt

Instructions

1. Add yoghurt and chlorella to a serving bowl. Stir until smooth.
2. Top with banana, figs, pine nuts, and salt, then enjoy.

Overnight Vanilla Vitality Oatmeal

Serves 1

- 2 tablespoons raisins
- 1 tablespoon hemp hearts
- 1 tablespoon flax seeds
- ½ cup gluten-free oats
- ¼ teaspoon ground cinnamon
- 1 pinch sea salt
- 1 cup unsweetened kefir (dairy or dairy-free)
- ¼ teaspoon pure vanilla extract
- 1 tablespoon raw honey

Instructions

1. Add all ingredients to a large mason jar. Stir to combine, then seal with a lid.
2. Refrigerate overnight. Enjoy the next morning.

Get-Ready Greens A.M. Skillet

Serves 1

- 1 tablespoon coconut oil
- 1 small yam, peeled and diced
- 1 scallion, chopped
- 1 cup shredded kale
- ½ cup broth
- ½ a 15-oz BPA-free can lentils, drained and rinsed
- 2 tablespoons goat cheese (or dairy-free cheese)
- 1 dash kelp sprinkles

Instructions

1. Omnivore Option: Sub ½ cup diced smoked salmon for the lentils

2. Add oil to a medium skillet over medium heat. When hot, add yam, scallion, and kale. Cook for 5 minutes or until golden brown.
3. Add broth. Cover and reduce heat to maintain a gentle simmer for 8 minutes or until sweet potatoes tender.
4. Stir in lentils to heat through. Serve topped with cheese and kelp.

Smoothie Power

Serves 1

- 1 ½ cups milk (dairy or dairy-free)
- 1 cup baby spinach
- 1 cup chopped romaine
- 1 small avocado
- 1 green apple, cored and chopped
- 1 small frozen banana
- 2 scoops vanilla protein powder
- 1 teaspoon spirulina powder
- 1 dash kelp sprinkles

Instructions

1. Add all ingredients to a high-speed blender. Blend until smooth.

Snacks

Sweet & Sour Kale Chips

Serves 2

- 1 bunch kale
- ½ tablespoon coconut oil, melted
- ½ tablespoon maple syrup
- ½ tablespoon raw apple cider vinegar
- 1 dash garlic powder
- Sea salt and black pepper, to taste

Instructions

1. Heat oven to 275 degrees F. Remove the rib and centre stem from the kale leaves. Cut kale into about 2-inch pieces.
2. In a large mixing bowl, toss kale in coconut oil to coat. Add maple syrup, vinegar, and dry seasonings over the top, then toss again to coat well.
3. Bake for about 20 minutes, turning kale over halfway through baking time. Watch for pieces to

dry out and remove smaller pieces as they get done. You want the chips to be slightly brown on the edges and crispy.

4. Serve immediately and enjoy!

Maca Tahini Fig Bites

Makes 12 bites

- 1 ½ cups dried figs, soaked in hot water for 30 minutes
- ½ cup unsweetened tahini
- 3 tablespoons coconut oil
- 1 tsp pure vanilla extract
- ¼ cup toasted sesame seeds
- ¼ teaspoon coarse sea salt

Instructions

1. Drain the figs very well, then remove any stems. Add figs, tahini, coconut oil, and vanilla to a food processor, then puree until smooth.

2. Transfer mixture to a loaf pan lined with parchment paper. Press the mixture down flat. Sprinkle sesame seeds and salt over the top.
3. Cover the pan, then place in the fridge to chill for 6 hours or until very firm, Slice into 12 squares, then enjoy!

Lunchtime

Hummus Veggie Collard Wrap

Serves 2

- 2 large collard leaves
- 1 cup roasted red pepper hummus
- 1 large avocado, sliced
- ¼ small red onion, thinly sliced
- 1 small cucumber, thinly sliced
- 1 tomato, thinly sliced
- 1 cup sprouts
- Sea salt and black pepper, to taste
- 1 dash kelp sprinkles
- 2.5 oz sweet potato chips cooked in coconut oil

Instructions

1. OMNIVORE OPTION: Add 4 slices of nitrate-free turkey to each wrap before rolling up.
2. Lay collard leaves on a flat surface. Layer hummus, avocado, onion, cucumber, tomato, and sprouts. Season with salt and pepper.
3. Roll them up like burritos, then slice them in half diagonally. Serve chips on the side.

Raspberry Lime Kale Salad

Serves 2

- 1 cup shredded kale
- Juice of 1 large lime
- 1 15-oz BPA-free can chickpeas, drained and rinsed
- 2 cups shredded purple cabbage
- ½ cup shredded carrots
- 1 large red bell pepper, very thinly sliced
- 1 scallion, thinly sliced
- 1 large avocado, chopped
- Sea salt and black pepper, to taste

- ¼ cup raw pumpkin seeds
- 1 cup raspberries
- ¼ cup cultured vegetables

Instructions

1. OMNIVORE OPTION: Top the prepared salads each with 5 oz BPA-free canned wild salmon in water (drained and flaked).
2. Add kale and lime juice to a large mixing bowl. Massage well with your hands until kale is wilted.
3. Add all remaining ingredients. Toss gently to combine, then allow to rest and marinate for about 15 minutes before serving.

Garden Enchantress Salad

Serves 2

- 3 cups baby spinach
- 3 cups chopped romaine
- 1 cucumber, chopped
- 1 small green bell pepper, chopped
- 2 tablespoons fresh parsley, chopped
- 1 cup broccoli florets, chopped

- 1 avocado, chopped
- ¼ cup plain yoghourt (dairy or dairy-free)
- 1 tablespoon raw honey
- ½ tablespoon herbs de Provence
- Sea salt and black pepper, to taste
- 4 hard-boiled eggs, chopped
- 1 scallion, thinly sliced

Instructions

1. OMNIVORE OPTION: Top prepared salads each with 3 oz cooked, peeled, and chilled shrimp.
2. Add all ingredients (except eggs and scallion) to a large mixing bowl. Toss gently to combine, then divide between two serving bowls.
3. Top salads with eggs and scallion, then enjoy.

Wise Woman Broccoli Soup

Serves 2

- 1 large sweet potato, roasted at 425 F until tender
- 3 cups broccoli florets, steamed
- 1 15-oz BPA-free can lentils, drained and rinsed

- 2 cups broth

- 1 cup milk (dairy or dairy-free)

- ½ teaspoon each garlic powder and onion powder

- Sea salt and black pepper, to taste

- 2 tablespoons minced chives

- 2 tablespoons plain yoghourt (dairy or dairy-free)

Instructions

1. OMNIVORE OPTION: Divide 4 slices of crispy chopped nitrate-free bacon or turkey bacon on top of the prepared soups.

2. Cool the roasted sweet potato slightly, then peel and dice it. Add diced sweet potato, steamed broccoli, lentils, broth, milk, and dry seasonings to a medium pot over medium heat.

3. Bring to a simmer, then remove from the heat. Carefully use an immersion blender in the pot OR transfer the hot soup to a high-speed blender. Puree until very smooth.

4. Pour into serving bowls, then top with chives.

Apple Jar Salad

Serves 2

- 1 small red apple, cored and diced
- 1 small green apple, cored and diced
- 2 tablespoons extra-virgin olive oil
- Juice of 1 lemon
- Sea salt and black pepper, to taste
- 1 cup cauliflower florets, chopped
- 1 15-oz BPA-free can black beans, drained and rinsed
- ½ cup shredded carrots
- ½ cup radishes, diced
- 1 red bell pepper, chopped
- 4 cups arugula
- ¼ cup raw pumpkin seeds

Instructions

1. OMNIVORE OPTION: Top the prepared salads each with 5 oz BPA-free canned tuna in water (drained and flaked).

2. Divide and layer ingredients in order listed between two 4-cup mason jars. Seal, then store in the fridge until ready to serve.
3. To serve, shake the sealed jars gently to disperse the dressing. Enjoy straight from the jars or pour into serving bowls.

Dinnertime

Ready-to-go Root Bowls

Serves 4

Roots

- 2 large sweet potatoes peeled and large-chopped
- 1 large rutabaga, peeled and large-chopped
- 1 large carrot, peeled and large-chopped
- 2 large turnips, peeled and large-chopped
- 1 large beet, peeled and large-chopped
- 2 tablespoons coconut oil, melted
- Sea salt and black pepper, to taste
- 1 teaspoon dried dill
- 1 teaspoon garlic powder

- 2 15-ounce BPA-free can chickpeas, drained and rinsed

Bowls

- 8 cups arugula
- 2 large tomatoes, large-chopped
- 2 scallions, thinly sliced
- 1 cup cultured vegetables

Instructions

1. OMNIVORE OPTION: Top the prepared bowls each with ½ cup shredded meat from a deli roast chicken.
2. Heat oven to 425 F. Line a large sheet pan with parchment. Add all ROOTS ingredients to the sheet pan, then use tongs to toss.
3. Spread out into an even layer. Bake for 50 minutes, tossing halfway through cooking time, or until tender.
4. Divide arugula between 4 serving bowls. Divide the ROOTS mixture on top of the arugula. Top with tomatoes, scallions, and cultured vegetables.

Vitality Sheet Pan Dinner

Serves 4

- 3 cups cooked brown rice (prepared to package instructions)
- 2 large zucchini, chopped
- 2 pounds asparagus, tough ends trimmed and discarded
- 2 large yellow bell peppers, chopped
- 2 cup cherry tomatoes
- 1 large yellow onion, halved and sliced
- 3 cloves garlic, chopped
- 2 tablespoons coconut oil, melted
- Juice of 1 large lemon
- 1 ½ tablespoons Italian seasoning
- Sea salt and black pepper, to taste
- ½ teaspoon crushed red pepper (optional)
- 2 15-oz BPA-free cans white kidney beans

Instructions

1. OMNIVORE OPTION: Add 1 lb whole boneless skinless chicken thighs on top of the tossed vegetables before baking.

2. Preheat the oven to 400 degrees F. Line a large sheet pan with parchment paper, then add all ingredients (except beans) to the pan. Use tongs to toss, then spread veggies out in an even layer.

3. Bake for 45 minutes, tossing halfway through cooking time with tongs, or until veggies are tender. Remove sheet pan from the oven, then stir in the beans. Bake for 5 more minutes to allow beans to heat through.

4. Serve the sheet pan mixture on top of cooked brown rice.

Quinoa Turmeric Skillet

Serves 4

- 2 tablespoons coconut oil
- 2 cups frozen chopped bell peppers and onions mix
- 4 cups cauliflower florets
- 1 cup shredded carrots
- 1 cup frozen green peas
- Sea salt and black pepper, to taste
- ½ teaspoon ground turmeric
- 1 teaspoon ground ginger

- ½ teaspoon garlic powder
- ½ teaspoon ground cinnamon
- 2 15-oz BPA-free cans chickpeas, drained and rinsed
- ¼ cup raisins
- 1 ½ cups dry quinoa
- 3 cups broth
- ½ cup chopped cilantro
- 1 large lime, sliced into 8 wedges

Instructions

1. OMNIVORE OPTION: Crumble in 1 pound ground beef after sautéing the bell peppers and onions.
2. Add oil to a large skillet over medium heat. When hot, add frozen mix and cauliflower. Cover and cook for about 5 minutes or until slightly tender.
3. Stir in carrots, peas, dry seasonings, chickpeas, raisins, quinoa, and broth. Cover and reduce heat to medium-low. Cook for 15 to 20 minutes or until the quinoa has absorbed all broth.
4. Serve topped with cilantro and with lime wedges on the side.

Sushi Burger Wraps

Serves 4

Sushi Mayo

- ¼ cup organic soy-free mayonnaise
- 1 tablespoon Sriracha (optional)
- 2 teaspoons coconut aminos
- 1 teaspoon toasted sesame oil

Burgers

- 4 soy-free veggie burger patties
- 4 large green leaf lettuce leaves
- 2 avocados, sliced
- 1 large cucumber, thinly sliced
- 1 cup sprouts

To Serve

- 2 cups radishes, thinly sliced
- 4 5-gram packages roasted seaweed in avocado oil (like GimMe Organic)

Instructions

1. OMNIVORE OPTION: Use cooked ground turkey patties in place of veggie patties
2. Add all SUSHI MAYO ingredients to a small mixing bowl. Whisk until smooth, then set aside.
3. Prepare burger patties according to package directions, then set aside.
4. Divide lettuce leaves flat between 4 serving plates. Spread leaves with SUSHI MAYO, then top them with avocados, cucumber, sprouts, and cooked burger patties. Fold the lettuce leaves over the ingredients to create wraps.
5. Serve with sliced radishes and seaweed on the side.

Paella Pasta

Serves 4

- 12 oz package chickpea pasta, cooked to package directions
- 2 tablespoons coconut oil
- 1 cup frozen diced onions
- 2 large yellow bell peppers, diced
- 1 cup frozen green peas
- 1 15-oz BPA-free can crushed tomatoes

- Juice of 1 lemon
- 1 15-oz BPA-free can black beans, drained and rinsed
- 1 teaspoon ground cumin
- 1 teaspoon ground paprika
- Sea salt and black pepper, to taste
- ½ cup chopped parsley

Large Salad

- 6 cups mixed greens
- 1 large tomato, chopped
- 1 large cucumber, chopped
- ¼ small red onion, sliced
- ¼ cup extra virgin olive oil
- 3 tablespoons balsamic vinegar
- 1 tablespoon raw honey
- Sea salt and black pepper, to taste

Instructions

1. OMNIVORE OPTION: Sub 1 lb raw, cleaned and peeled shrimp plus ½ lb raw baby scallops for the black beans.
2. Prepare the pasta and set aside.
3. Heat oil in a large pot over medium heat. When hot, add onion and bell peppers. Cook for 8 minutes, stirring occasionally, until tender.
4. Stir in all remaining ingredients (except parsley). Cook, stirring occasionally, for 10 minutes or until thickened. Stir in cooked pasta to heat through.
5. Serve topped with parsley. Toss all LARGE SALAD ingredients in a large bowl, then serve salads on the side.

Desserts

Cacao Hemp Pudding

Serves 2

- ½ cup chia seeds
- ¼ cup hemp hearts
- 3 tablespoons raw cacao powder
- ½ teaspoon pure vanilla extract
- 1 pinch sea salt

- ¼ cup maple syrup
- 1 cup milk (dairy or dairy-free)

Instructions

1. Add all ingredients to a high-speed blender. Blend on low speed until the cacao is dissolved.
2. Pour into two serving bowls. Cover and chill in the fridge for 4 hours or until fully set.

18. Menopause Resources and Links

1. Menopause.org - https://www.menopause.org/
2. YogaPauseTV - https://www.youtube.com/@yogapausetv
3. The Pink Table Podcast - https://podcasters.spotify.com/pod/show/yogabellies
4. The Hormone Health Network - https://www.hormone.org/your-health-and-hormones/womens-health/menopause
5. The Menopause Movement - https://www.menopausemovement.com/
6. Menopause Goddess Blog - https://www.menopausegoddessblog.com/
7. Women's Health Concern - https://www.womens-health-concern.org/
8. Healthline Menopause - https://www.healthline.com/health/menopause
9. My Menopause Magazine - https://www.mymenopausemagazine.com/
10. The Menopause Exchange - https://www.menopause-exchange.co.uk/

11. Menopause Chicks - https://www.menopausechicks.com/
12. Menopause Support - https://www.menopausesupport.org.uk/
13. Red Hot Mamas - https://redhotmamas.org/
14. The Menopause Doctor - https://menopausedoctor.co.uk/
15. The Vagina Dialogues - https://www.thevaginadialogues.com/
16. Menopause Goddesses Facebook Group - https://www.facebook.com/groups/menopausegoddesses/
17. The Menopause Coach Facebook Group - https://www.facebook.com/groups/themenopausecoach/
18. The Perimenopause Hub Facebook Group - https://www.facebook.com/groups/perimenopausehub/
19. The Menopause Cafe - https://www.menopausecafe.net/
20. Menopause Sisters - https://www.menopausesisters.com/
21. Menopause Matters - https://www.menopausematters.co.uk/

22. The Menopause Mindset Summit - https://www.menopausemindsetsummit.com/

Bibliography

Avis, N. E., Crawford, S. L., & McKinlay, S. M. (1997). Psychosocial, behavioural, and health factors related to menopause symptomatology. *Women's Health, 3*(2), 103-120.

Bahri, S., & Zargar, A. H. (2016). Nutritional management of menopausal symptoms. *Journal of Mid-life Health, 7*(4), 171-173.

Beepollenhub. (2015). *Bee pollen and menopause - Basic information.* http://www.beepollenhub.com/bee-pollen-and-menopause/

Bijlani, R. L., Vempati, R. P., Yadav, R. K., Ray, R. B., Gupta, V., Sharma, R., ... & Mahapatra, S. C. (2005). A brief but comprehensive lifestyle education program based on yoga reduces risk factors for cardiovascular disease and diabetes mellitus. *Journal of Alternative and Complementary Medicine, 11*(2), 267-274.

Bock, B. C., Fava, J. L., Gaskins, R. B., Morrow, K. M., Williams, D. M., Jennings, E., ... & Marcus, B. H. (2014). Yoga as a complementary therapy for smoking cessation in women. *Journal of Women's Health, 23*(10), 824-831.

Brighten, J. (2023). *15 perimenopause supplements for happy hormones.* https://drbrighten.com/perimenopause-supplements/

Calasanti, T. M., & King, N. (2007). Ageism and feminism: From "et cetera" to centre. *NWSA Journal, 19*(2), 13-30.

Chattha, R., Raghuram, N., Venkatram, P., & Hongasandra, N.R. (2008). Treating the climacteric symptoms in Indian women with an integrated approach to yoga therapy: A randomized control study. *Menopause, 15*(5), 862-870.

Chen, M. N., Lin, C. C., & Liu, C. F. (2016). Efficacy of phytoestrogens for menopausal symptoms: A meta-analysis and systematic review. *Climacteric, 19*(2), 125-135.

Chittister, J. (2008). The gift of years: Growing older gracefully. Bluebridge.

Chong, C. S., Tsunaka, M., Tsang, H. W., Chan, E. P., & Cheung, W. M. (2011). Effects of yoga on stress management in healthy adults: A systematic review. *Alternative Therapies in Health and Medicine, 17*(1), 32-38.

Compagine Cohen, A. (2021). *Progesterone and perimenopause: What you need to know.* https://well.org/?s=Progesterone+and+Perimenopause%3A+What+You+Need+to+Know

Cruikshank, M. (2003). Feminist gerontology and old men. *Journal of Aging Studies, 17*(1), 59-73.

Domes, G., Heinrichs, M., Michel, A., Berger, C., & Herpertz, S. C. (2007). Oxytocin improves "mind-reading" in humans. *Biological Psychiatry, 61*(6), 731-733.

Faubion, S.S. (2018). Mayo Clinic the perimenopause solution: A doctor's guide to relieving hot flashes, enjoying better sex, sleeping well, controlling your weight, and being happy! TI Inc Books.

Flo. (2023). *8 natural supplements for perimenopause.* https://flo.health/menstrual-cycle/menopause/symptoms/supplements-for-perimenopause

Francina, S. (2003) Yoga and the wisdom of menopause: A guide to physical, emotional and spiritual health at midlife and beyond. Health Communications, Inc.

Francina, S. (2004) Yoga for menopause: Safe and effective practice for a healthy transition. Health Communications, Inc.

Frankel, L. (2004). Ageless women, timeless wisdom: Witty, wicked, and wise reflections on well-lived lives. Skyhorse.

Friedman, H.S., & Martin, L.R. (2012). The longevity project: Surprising discoveries for health and long life from the landmark eight-decade study. Plume.

Gallegos, A. M., Hoerger, M., Talbot, N. L., Moynihan, J. A., & Duberstein, P. R. (2013). Emotional benefits of mindfulness-based stress reduction in older adults: The moderating role of age and depressive symptom severity. *Aging & Mental Health, 17*(7), 823-829.

Garrett, A. (2019). Perimenopause: The savvy sister's guide to hormone harmony. Anna Garrett Companies LLC.

Gittleman, A.L. (2001). Before the change: Taking charge of your perimenopause. HarperOne.

Gold, E. B., Colvin, A., Avis, N., Bromberger, J., Greendale, G. A., Powell, L., ... & Matthews, K. (2006). Longitudinal analysis of the association between vasomotor symptoms and race/ethnicity across the menopausal transition: Study of women's health across the nation. *American Journal of Public Health, 96*(7), 1226-1235.

Good Health. (2023). *The adrenal connection with menopause.* https://www.goodhealth.co.nz/health-articles/article/the-adrenal-connection-with-menopause#:~:text=The%20connection%20betwe en%20adrenals%20and,take%20over%20female%20 hormonal%20production

Goodsell, L. (2019). *Yoga for pregnancy.* https://mandalabirthing.com/yoga-for-pregnancy/

Grewen, K. M., Davenport, R. E., & Light, K. C. (2010). An investigation of plasma and salivary oxytocin responses in breast- and formula-feeding mothers of infants. *Psychophysiology, 47*(4), 625-632.

Gwen. (2022). The perimenopause diet: 15 foods to eat and avoid. *Meraki Lane*. https://www.merakilane.com/the-perimenopause-diet-15-foods-to-eat-and-avoid/

Hale, S. (2023). *Progesterone during pregnancy: Uses & treatments. Miracare* https://www.miracare.com/blog/progesterone-during-pregnancy/

Hunter, M. (2015). The South-East England longitudinal study of the climacteric and postmenopause. *Climacteric, 18*(1), 15-22.

Indiana University. (2023). *National survey of sexual health and behavior.* https://nationalsexstudy.indiana.edu/

Innes, K.E., Selfe, T.K., & Vishnu, A. (2010). Mind-body therapies for menopausal symptoms: A systematic review. *Maturitas, 66*(2), 135-149.

Khalsa, S. (2010). Yoga for women: Wellness and vitality at every stage of life. Dorling Kindersley Ltd.

Khalsa, S.B.S., & Faulkner, K.A. (2004). The effects of yoga on menopausal symptoms. *Menopause Management, 13*(3), 16-23.

Khoury, B., Sharma, M., Rush, S. E., & Fournier, C. (2015). Mindfulness-based stress reduction for healthy individuals: A meta-analysis. *Journal of Psychosomatic Research, 78*(6), 519-528.

Kinser, P. A., Bourguignon, C., Whaley, D., Hauenstein, E., & Taylor, A. G. (2013). Feasibility, acceptability, and effects of gentle Hatha yoga for women with major depression: Findings from a randomized controlled mixed-methods study. *Archives of Psychiatric Nursing, 27*(3), 137-147.

LaVoie, D. (2020). *The best superfoods for the menopause diet.* https://danalavoielac.com/the-best-superfoods-for-the-menopause-diet/

Live Well Zone. (2023). *Everything you need to know about estrogen dominance during perimenopause.* https://livewellzone.com/estrogen-dominance-during-perimenopause/

Mayo Clinic. (2021). *Perimenopause - Diagnosis and treatment.* https://www.mayoclinic.org/diseases-conditions/perimenopause/diagnosis-treatment/drc-20354671

Mayo Clinic. (2021). *Perimenopause - Symptoms and causes.* https://www.mayoclinic.org/diseases-conditions/perimenopause/symptoms-causes/syc-20354666

MenoLabs. (2020, October 21). How to know if you're in perimenopause. *Menolabs.* https://menolabs.com/blogs/menolife/how-to-know-if-youre-in-perimenopause

Menopause Now. (2019). *Perimenopause and hormones.* https://www.menopausenow.com/perimenopause/hormones

Migala, J. (2021, November 17). In your 40S? You'll want to add these 7 foods to your diet. *HUM.* https://www.humnutrition.com/blog/foods-for-perimenopause-diet/

Northrup, C. (2001). The wisdom of menopause: Creating physical and emotional health during the change. Bantam Books

Pascoe, M. C., & Bauer, I. E. (2015). A systematic review of randomised control trials on the effects of yoga on stress measures and mood. *Journal of Psychiatric Research, 68,* 270-282.

Petersson, M., Alster, P., Lundeberg, T., & Uvnäs-Moberg, K. (1998). Oxytocin causes a long-term decrease of blood pressure in female and male rats. *Physiology & Behavior, 63*(3), 381-387.

Pipher, M. (2019). Women rowing north: Navigating life's currents and flourishing as we age. Bloomsbury Publishing.

Prima. (2016, April 27). The 34 symptoms of perimenopause you need to know. *Prima.* https://www.prima.co.uk/diet-and-health/news/a35329/perimenopause-pre-menopause-recognise-symptoms/

Rittenhouse, M., & Ozawa, M. N. (2016). Resisting ageism through feminist gerontology. *Journal of Women & Aging, 28*(6), 490-502.

Rosenblatt, J. S. (2014). Oxytocin and maternal behavior. In D. Pfaff & M. Joels (Eds.), *Hormones, brain and behavior* (3rd ed., pp. 249-274). Elsevier.

Ruan, X., Jin, Y., Kato, H., Amakawa, T., & Yamamoto, Y. (2017). The relationship between dietary intake and menopausal symptoms in Chinese women: A cross-sectional study. *Journal of Obstetrics and Gynaecology Research, 43*(1), 168-174.

Russell, M. (2012). Menopause yoga: A guide to practise, a guide to wellness.

Santoro, N., & Randolph, J. F. Jr. (2011). Reproductive hormones and the menopause transition. *Obstetrics and Gynecology Clinics, 38*(3), 455-466.

Santosa, S., & Demonty, I. (2017). Inflammation and menopause: A narrative review. *Journal of Women's Health, 26*(6), 553-559.

Shantakumari, N., Sequeira, S., & Deeb R. (2013). Effects of a yoga intervention on lipid profiles of diabetes patients with dyslipidemia. *Indian Heart Journal, 65*(2), 127-131.

SheCares. (2020). *Progesterone and menopause.* https://www.shecares.com/hormones/progesterone/menopause

Snowdon, D. (2002). *More meaningful lives.* Bantam Press.

Snyder, M. (2019). The best essential oils for perimenopause. *MBG Health.* https://www.mindbodygreen.com/articles/best-essential-oils-for-perimenopause

Sontag, S. (1972). The double standard of ageing. *The Saturday Review,* 55-60.

Todd, N. (2022). *Ways your vagina changes as you age.* https://www.webmd.com/women/ss/slideshow-ways-your-vagina-changes-as-you-age#:~:text=Just%20like%20the%20rest%20of,at%20this%20stage%20of%20life

Twigg, J. (2004). The body, gender, and age: Feminist insights in social gerontology. *Journal of Aging Studies, 18*(1), 59-73.

Uvnäs-Moberg, K., & Petersson, M. (2005). Oxytocin, a mediator of anti-stress, well-being, social interaction, growth and healing. *Zeitschrift Für Psychosomatische Medizin Und Psychotherapie, 51*(1), 57-80.

Velez, A. (2017, December 1). Do you have adrenal fatigue or perimenopause? *Prevention*. https://www.prevention.com/health/a20509002/adrenal-fatigue-or-perimenopause/

Woods, N. F., Mitchell, E. S., & Smith-DiJulio, K. (2009). Menopause symptom clusters and their relationship to women's health and psychosocial status. *Menopause, 16*(2), 399-408.

Yang, Y., Kim, S., & Kim, J. (2016). The effects of a yoga program on women's menstrual cycle and symptoms. *Journal of Alternative and Complementary Medicine, 22*(4), 324-331.

About the Author

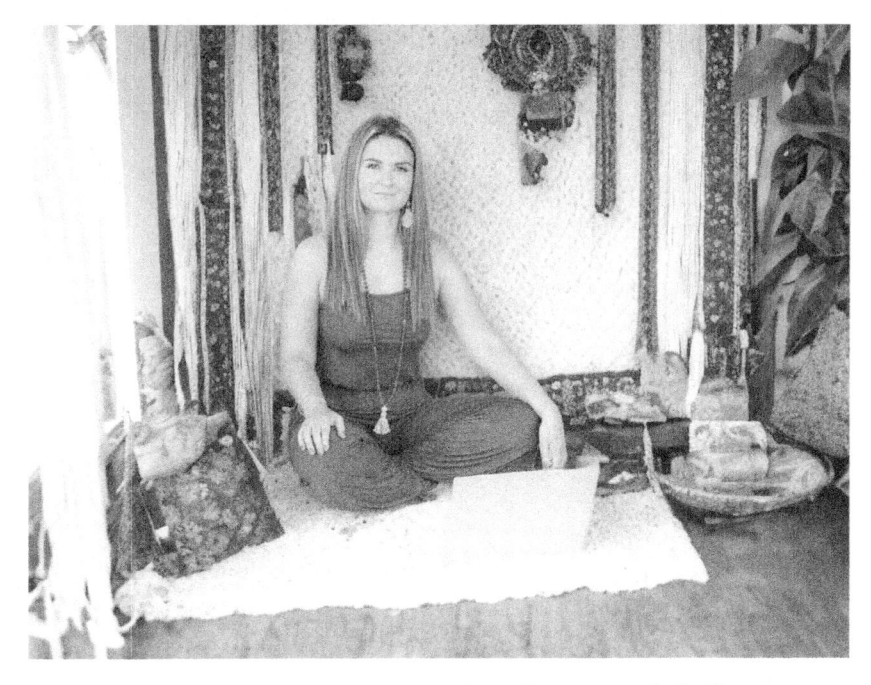

Cheryl Kennedy MacDonald is a celebrity yoga teacher, an author and even a Dragons' Den winner! Cheryl created YogaBellies as an inclusive community for women. Using yoga as a platform for support, health and wellness for women at every life stage. Cheryl started teaching pregnancy yoga classes from home and things grew very quickly from there. YogaBellies now has hundreds of teachers across the world teaching the YogaBellies and YogaPause methods. She's the author of several best-selling books about yoga and women's health and spends her time hosting retreats and training yoga teachers across the world. Cheryl currently lives in Singapore with her son, Caelen and her husband Mike, a Cardiologist. Find out more about YogaBellies or YogaPause at www.yogabellies.com and follow Cheryl on Instagram @yogabellies @cherylyogabellies. You can also check out The Pink Table Podcast or YogaBelliesTV and YogaPauseTV on YouTube.

Love this book? Check out the accompanying journal

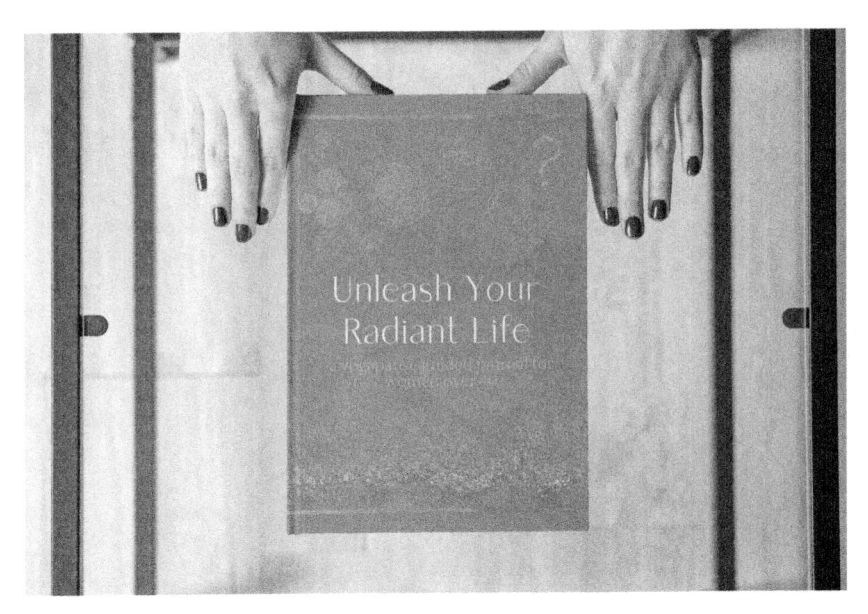

Unleashing Your Radiant Life: A YogaPause Guided Journal For Women Over 40

The "Unleashing Your Radiant Life journal" is a transformative companion journal to the YogaPause book. As we transition into the Enchantress and Wise Woman stages of life, this phase often invites us to explore the full spectrum of our lives—intellectual and spiritual growth, family and relationships, house & home, health & fitness, adventures, career, and finances.

YogaPause

This journal offers a unique opportunity for introspection and clarity. It prompts you to crystalize what truly matters and envision the life you want to lead going forward and track your menopause journey.

[Buy it now on Amazon](#)

Printed in Great Britain
by Amazon